Second Chance

Regain Your Health With Tissue Salts

by

Eva F. Schoenfeld

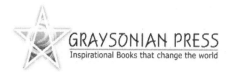

GRAYSONIAN PRESS
Inspirational Books that change the world

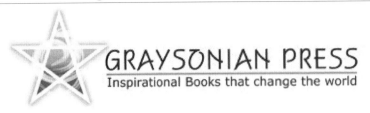

GRAYSONIAN PRESS
Inspirational Books that change the world

Published by Graysonian Press www.graysonian.com pat@graysonian.com
+27 11 6462956

Printed in South Africa

Cover designed by: Tim Morrison of Ink Pot Designs
Edited by Lia Schurman

ISBN 978-0-620-43937-4

Biography

Eva F. Schoenfeld was born in Switzerland 1945. She has a degree in Business Management and successfully operated her own Event Organization company running major Sport-Events.

Due to health problems, she started studying different healing arts. This led her on a path where she studied in Switzerland, Germany, Austria and the USA. She also practiced what she learnt in holistic centers (not only on human beings, but also animals) in Switzerland, Germany and Spain. She is a Facial Analyst & Tissue Salt Consultant (Biochemistry), Jin Shin Jyutsu® Practitioner, Esalen® Massage Practitioner and Reiki Master and teacher.

Since 2005 she has lived in South Africa where she runs the Academy of Tissue Salts and Facial Analysis.

Referring to Tissue Salts, Eva tells as many people as possible, 'they saved my life', and so her passion for the salts led her to help hundreds of clients. It was this same passion that inspired her to write this book, as she wants to tell as many people as possible about the amazing healing affects of Tissue Salts.

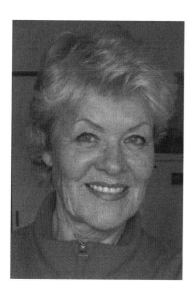

Acknowledgments

I wish to express my gratitude to Thomas Feichtinger (Biochemical Association Austria), the real father of this book. He taught me about Tissue Salts and Facial Analysis. I thank him for his contribution.

Foreword

Driven by her passion to help as many as possible, and inspired by what she, herself had had learnt of the value of this system of therapeutics, Eva F. Schoenfeld was motivated to write this inspiring treatise on Nature's dynamic healing remedies, the biochemical Tissue Salts, as introduced to the world by the creative genius of Dr W H Schuessler.

Every one of these inorganically sourced remedies is supplied in organic and natural state and form in the vegetables and fruit we eat. Also they are natural and essential constituents of the normal, healthy growth and life of organic beings. But, as Eva so eloquently discusses - in our present day exposure we have to live in an environment which is virtually and almost universally contaminated. By having to depend for our nourishment upon foods grown in soils rendered nutrient deficient, it is almost inevitable that we will experience dis-ease, disabilities and a whole gamut of psychosomatic ailments.

Not only do the twelve essential Tissue Salts treat and benefit the body with their biochemical healing properties; when correctly manufactured (according to the strict and precise requirements of homoeopathic trituration), they also contain the homeopathically produced vibrational quantum energy embedded in them. This time and effort demanding pharmaceutical operation may legitimately be executed only by manufacturers approved by the South Africa's Medicines Control Council.

Dr. Michael Levien DH, ND, DO
Registered Phytotherapist and Ayurvedic Practitioner.

Introduction - Dream a little

Imagine waking up early each morning with your mind as clear as a mountain stream, a mind that can't wait to get out of bed to conquer and achieve all that it sets its sights on.

You go to the bathroom, and see a face that's smooth and unblemished, it has no wrinkles of worry or abuse. Your eyes glow with life and shine with excitement. You've only been awake for five minutes but feel the exuberance of a four year old and want to run and hop.

Hours have gone by and you are in the later part of the work day. The time passes quickly as you eat up the demands that your job entails. Your memory is good and wit lightening sharp.

Once back at home, there is no need to lounge about in a mindless fog while your energy struggles to catch up after the demands of the day. Full of bounce, you and the dogs canter around the streets, whilst appreciating the green gardens of your neighbourhood.

Later, the brain processes, absorbs and categorises your latest study project. The spring in your step is as elastic and lively as it was 17 hours before when you exploded out of bed.

Does a life like this sound too good to be true? At the start of this short piece, I asked you to dream a little. This dream that you just had can become real for you. Read on and see how Tissue Salts can help you create that dream…

What you will find in this book

This book tells you what tissue salts are and how they work. To support this; there are case studies, photos showing facial symptoms, a psychosomatic profiling for people with Tissue Salt deficiencies and a handy A to Z of complaints with over 700 symptoms and treatments using tissue salts.

Publishers note
Whilst editing this book, every effort has been made to preserve the voice of Eva, that is, one of a Swiss speaking nationalist, writing in a second language.

Synopsis

Dr Wilhelm Schuessler, a German medical doctor and homeopath, rediscovered (over 130 years ago) that mineral substances have a major job to do for the body. He diluted, and thus miniaturised them to become sufficiently small and delicate enough for their easy acceptance into the human cellular system. Once absorbed, they perform their daily labour for the entire organism. Without these fine-tuned helpers we could become ill and die - they are absolutely vital for ongoing life. Dr Schuessler called his discovery Biochemistry.

Mankind has used Dr Schuessler's mineral substances for more than 100 years to the welfare and benefit of a well-functioning body. These mineral substances were described in Sanskrit, which demonstrates that the significance of an adequate availability of body-own mineral substances had already earned recognition at that time.

Depleted and over fertilised soil

In Dr Schuessler's time, depleted and over fertilised soil was not an issue and people obtained their minerals through normal nourishment. Unfortunately this situation has drastically changed over the years, where our soils have become mineral deficient.

Our parents and grandparents all aged without having heard of Schuessler salts. But the culmination and the effects of the toxin exposure we have had over the last 20 years or so are now coming to the fore. Now, more than ever Dr Schuessler's Tissue Salts are imperative as a major factor to stem this destructive trend in our bodies. In the past there was not much need for the salts, but now, they are absolutely essential as a survival factor.

Vitamin and supplements

For some time people have held the ill-informed belief that minerals can (on the cellular level) be replaced by vitamins and nutritional supplements. Little do they know that vitamins and supplements can only get cellular acceptance if the cells are adequately mineral-enriched. A cellular balance is first required. If these minerals (Tissue Salts) are absent, the body will battle to absorb even a tiny fraction of these intruders. This becomes a stress factor for the cells.

Facial analysis

Dr Schuessler discovered that mineral deficiencies present themselves as discolorations, shadows, wrinkles and furrows in the face. He understood facial analysis as an art, and for him, all these signs were clear indications of an impending disorder. The signs of deficiencies are easy to learn and can be used by everybody. These signs are described in this manual. Disorders can also be easily corrected at an early stage by administering the right Tissue Salts blend.

Psychosomatic considerations

As biochemistry knowledge progressed, Schuessler's successors discovered that mineral deficiencies also have psychosomatic connections. Certain human behaviour patterns demonstrate specific deficiencies and vice versa. As minerals do their work on the cellular level they are capable of altering the cell information. With this discovery, a new understanding and awareness came into being about restoring and maintaining, not only excellent health, but also to gain a long-term influence over certain obsessive behaviour patterns!

Table of content

About Tissue Salts

Tissue Salts, also known as cell salts or biochemistry salts, are the same minerals that are found in rocks and soil. They also occur naturally in the human body. In the past, lost or used body minerals could easily be replaced through normal nutrition. But today's 'empty' food harvested from nutritionally drained soil leads to constant mineral depletion.

We also lose minerals through stress, worry, fast life styles, bad nutrition, industrially tainted foodstuffs, electro-pollution, (cell phones, microwaves, computers), and through environmental toxins (insecticides, pesticides, preservatives, etc), as well as exposure to heavy metals, such as amalgam dental fillings, lead, aluminium, contaminated drinking water ... the list could go on endlessly.

In fact, because the missing minerals are not being replaced, it appears as if humanity is becoming weaker and more disease-prone from generation to generation. This tendency is very much in evidence - if we only consider the worrisome increase in babies that are born with allergies and other deficiencies as a result of a mineral deficiency within the mother. What the mother lacked in minerals during pregnancy, the child will be lacking at birth. This is one of the reasons for the ongoing and increasing generational deficiencies. Until mankind accepts the policy of a regular mineral replacement, the deficiencies will continue to escalate. However, with the application of the correct amount of Tissue Salts, the body can heal and restore itself from within.

The three main principles of Schuessler's thesis are:

• The human body contains 12 vital mineral salts, which need to be properly balanced for normal health

• When this balance is disturbed, disease follows

• The balance can easily be re-established by administering the deficient mineral salts in a readily assimilated form. The most effective of which is a triturated form (Tissue Salts).

Tissue Salts are essential biochemical function agents. When mineral-deficient, we feel tired, exhausted and suffer from skin, hair or nail problems. We feel sluggish and do not look well.

Show me your face – and I'll tell you what you are lacking!

That of course is a very risky sentence – but true! The face reveals mineral deficiencies in different ways. A trained practitioner can detect many body complaints, but I am ahead of myself.

Many years ago, because of my own complaints, I gained knowledge in the art of Facial Analysis. For several years I lived in a house with lots of electro pollution and field lines (radiation). What I didn't know about radiation was that because of it, the body needed lots of minerals to restore functionality. I was exhausted and had no power or vitality. Not knowing what was wrong with me, I went to a doctor. Of course, he couldn't find anything wrong. But even so, he wanted to give me antibiotics – just in case I had a virus. Of course, I refused the antibiotics.

A few weeks later, I discovered Dr Schuessler's Tissue Salts. A friend of mine had the salts and suggested that I take some. Not knowing about them, I simply took a handful of each number and sucked them. Half an hour later, I had an incredible experience; my whole body became totally relaxed, I could breathe deeply and felt much better. Wow! Of course I wanted to know more about Tissue Salts. A week later I registered for the first of many workshops, where I learnt about Biochemistry, Tissue Salts and Facial Analysis. Professionally supported and advised, I continued taking the salts and gradually regained my health and vitality, and so can you!

I was already a professional caregiver using Esalen® Massage, Body working, Reflexology, Reiki and Jin Shin Jyutsu®. But once I became a Tissue Salts consultant and Facial Analyst my patient success rate radically improved.

I was, and still am excited at the quick dynamic techniques of facial analysis for Tissue Salt deficiencies and how fast and easy the recovery from complaints is made possible, all by simply taking these precious minerals. I am simply no longer able to look at a face, as I am facinated to see any Tissue Salt deficiencies. Everyone, and especially all parents should understand about Tissue Salts for their children's requirements. By being able to do so they can prevent disturbances and maintain a good state of health.

Schuessler's discovery

Tissue Salts or Cell salts are vital mineral constituents of the body, where they combine with organic substances to produce and maintain the infinite number of tissue-cells of which the human body is composed. Thus, any cell salt deficiency or imbalance may result in illness, where the symptoms vary according to the deficient Biochemical Cell Salt. However, he went on to state that if the deficiency was corrected, the body could in fact heal itself.

Schuessler also discovered that if he gave the minerals in an undiluted or subdivided form they would not be able to enter the cells, and would also strain the organism. We know this effect from the usual (Macro) Calcium, Magnesium and Iron preparations. These should not be taken over an extended period, as they strain the body, resulting in undesirable side effects. If you have to take lots of Iron, your Zinc balance will be affected and the body will not be able to absorb Manganum and Selenium. Zinc is very important for wound healing, the building-up of sexual hormones, genes and proteins in the body. An imbalance is extremely detrimental, as the body cannot absorb Magnesium, Iron and Fluorine. The latest US-American research confirms that Women taking high doses of Calcium (600 mg) (after Menopause, in an effort to avoid Osteoporosis) can also develop a Zinc deficiency. An excessive intake of food-supplements (macro) like Selenium, Fluorine, Zinc, Vitamin A and D can be dangerous to your health. And here is an anomaly, we should be able to get all the necessary minerals and vitamins by eating healthy food, but we can't, as our food is barren.

Schuessler diluted the Tissues Salts so that they are able to penetrate through the minuscule apertures of the cell wall. This makes it impossible for anybody to take an overdose of these remedies.

However, to allay fears of overdosing on Tissue Salts, in a 1-liter-bottle of still mineral water there is an average of 100 mg of dissolved solids (minerals). If you were to take the same amount of Schuessler's Tissue Salts, you would have to dissolve 1-ton (1'000 kg) in the same size bottle! This shows the degree of dilution achieved by potency (dilution).

When Schuessler was alive, he was not confronted with depleted soils and industrially treated nutrition. Perhaps he already knew what we were to experience a hundred years later.

The effect of depleted soils

Once we recognise the effects of our depleted soil in South Africa, we will understand the regrettable occurrence of so many immune diseases in our country. The British Institute of Science in London has researched the mineral Selenium and discovered very interesting geographical connections. The research showed that the soil of the Southern Hemisphere is devoid of Zinc, Magnesium and Selenium. The latter being one of the most crucial natural immune boosters. They compared this to the North African country Senegal, where that country's soil is rich in Selenium. Immune diseases and many other ailments and are almost unknown there!

Recently the CSIRO (Commonwealth Scientific and Industrial Research Organisation) presented the results of their latest research of agrarian products in Australia. The test of the indigenous food confirmed that; there is a complete lack of Selenium in the grown food!

In China, the Selenium drained regions are very well known as illness belts.

These examples confirm the importance of supplementing Dr Schuessler's Tissue Salts as a replacement for missing minerals. No other product or method is as natural or as easily assimilated into the body's tissue.

Dr Schuessler discovered 12 different minerals in the human body. However, with continuing research, the Biochemical Associations in Europe discovered that the human body contains at least another 15 Tissue Salts. These are No13 to 27. Most support the body in its fight against the so-called "modern illnesses". No 26 Selenium, is the most important immune booster. No 21 Zincum muriaticum is considered as the 'brain-mineral'. Zinc, can be obtained in the Southern Hemisphere, but only if you eat seafood. Sadly this is usually contaminated with mercury.

The deplorable mineral deficiency which we have to live with negates the information supplied in all those wonderful books about nutrition, e.g. by Patrick Holford and many others. They quite correctly claim that you can improve your Magnesium and Zinc levels by eating Broccoli, or Spinach. But this is not valid for South Africa! Also, most of the supplements you get from health shops don't do the trick, simply because they either don't get absorbed into the blood stream. However, even if they did, the cells reject them, because of wrong artificial molecule size and as a result of the body being mineral-deficient (Tissue Salts)!

It is a good idea to buy organic vegetables, because organic farmers fertilise plantations with those minerals, which the plants suck in to transform into a palatable and absorbable form!

What are Tissue Salts?

Our parents and grandparents aged gracefully without taking Tissue Salts as there was simply no need. But with the culmination and the effects of toxin exposure, the effects exacerbated. It is for this reason why Tissue Salts are essentially a major factor to stem this destructive trend in our bodies. They are a necessary survival factor.

It is important to note that Schuessler's Tissue Salts:
• Are NOT drugs, but valuable micro dosed cell food, carefully prepared in an extremely subdivided form, which ensures rapid and easy assimilation, for the speedy restoration of the natural balance of the body system

• Are NON-habit-forming and have NO side effects, only reactions

• Can be applied to persons of any age, as well as to animals

• Are absolutely safe for children and pregnant woman.

The loss of minerals

Aggravating circumstances are; the pollution of our environment (which constantly increases), and the fact that our body depletes its deposit of mineral salts, simply to keep functioning. Not having sufficient natural minerals in our body leads to a loss of vitality, premature aging, over acidification, restrictions of mobility, allergies, which all can lead to diseases. As we feel more and more restricted on a physical level we can no longer take any kind of strain and our premature aging process becomes visible and perceptible (osteoporosis, problematic hair, fragile nails, weak skin, wrinkles, varicose veins etc.)

The main problem is one of not being able to replenish the minerals the body uses for its daily work. These results from the empty nutrition we get from barren soils. There are however, several other reasons for a loss of minerals, like Radiation (from Cell-phones, microwave, electromagnetic fields, computer's, etc.), heavy metal poisoning (such as amalgam fillings, cosmetics, insecticides, pesticides), nutrition (processed, refined and denaturised food), hyperacidity (soft drinks, too much meat), stress, lifestyle, drugs, etc.

Craving and Refusing

We also lose minerals due to cravings. Because Tissue Salts have a regulating effect, we need them if we crave for or refuse a food type. There is a link between someone who loves chocolate (and eats a lot of it) and a deficiency. This means there is a shortage in Magnesium on a cellular level (micro), and perhaps other minerals which result in the craving for chocolate. The assimilation and digestion of chocolate needs lots of Magnesium on a cellular level, thus more cravings occur. The more chocolate that is eaten, the bigger the deficiency in the cell. When one refills the shortage in the cells with the relevant Tissue Salts, the craving disappears.

You are in charge of what you put into your body!

Parents should not forget that they are in charge of what their children put in their bodies.

Holistic Health Components

Attitude

Attitude is crucial. If you are constantly negative and always finding fault (a pessimist), it will influence your entire system. The metabolism will slow down and energy level will lower, thereby attracting negativity. Conversely, when you are positive and optimistic you will find that you can deal more easily with difficult situations and they will not impact on your metabolism.

Energy fields

Often people try to improve their health, but fail to do so because of hidden energy fields. There are different kinds of energy fields, some of which I now describe.

Mirror radiation

Many people don't know the strain mirrors can cause, especially in the bedroom. The same for shiny surfaces (furniture, pictures), by reflecting the shiny rays in the room and reinforcing the existing energy fields (radiation). The energy field feels lighter after removing the mirror(s). Not everyone is sensitive enough to feel this, but many can. You will know only if you try it.

Electromagnetic fields

Electromagnetic fields are a big issue today as they are everywhere. It is almost daily that one reads about this negative energy, e.g. TV, remote controls, cell phones, laptops and computers, where they all emanate microwave radiation. You can't hear, smell or see radiation, but it is a fact – we are living under a tent of radiation. These appliances affect us in many ways. High-tension lines that are close to our homes are the cause of many health problems. The electromagnetic fields in concrete-metal-glass-buildings are extremely high and the body has to constantly fight its effects. It needs a lot of Tissue Salts to fight against electromagnetic radiation.

The reason why you get ill when you are exposed to radiation:
Every mineral has its own task. For example, one mineral is responsible for the working of the glands (No 5 Kalium muriaticum). If a person is exposed to radiation, the body needs to fight against the disturbance, which uses up this Tissue Salt. If the exposure is high and long, the need for this mineral becomes greater because there may be no working agents left for the detoxing and cleaning of the glands. If this is the case, the person will become more and more toxic. Only by refilling the deposits with the correct Tissue Salt and protecting it against radiation, will the body recover.

All kinds of electromagnetic fields have a huge influence on our body and cause a build up of acid. Cars and airplanes also have radiation. You probably know the exhausted feeling when you have driven or flown long distances. This is not jet-lag, as jet-lag is the result of moving through time zones.

To avoid this overtiredness whilst travelling, support the body's work by taking the following driver's mixture during your journey.

Drivers Mixture:

Ferr Phos No 4	10 tablets
Kali phos No 6	10 tablets
Kali sulf No 7	10 tablets
Nat mur No 9	10 tablets
Nat phos No 10	20 to 30 tablets
Nat sulf No 11	10 tablets

Put all the above tablets in a dish and shake well. Take the tablets one at a time, dissolving them in your mouth. You will arrive at your destination fresh and rested!

Bedroom

Having a TV in the bedroom or a computer can quadruple the electromagnetic strain! Very often the electric cables are installed adjacent to the bed where the head rests. Even when the lights or appliances are switched off, the strain is still there, as the electromagnetic fields remain constant. The result is that the body has to fight against this strain – whilst it is meant to rest and regenerate. The effect is that organisms don't detoxify and cause the waste to stay in the body. No wonder you wake up tired.

Kitchen

It is alarming to think that so many people use Microwave ovens.[3] The heating process heats the food from the inside and by doing so destroys the nutritional molecules. According to several scientific research projects, food prepared in Microwave ovens has a significant effect on the blood. In one test, 400 people were fed the same nutrition, 200 people ate it traditionally prepared, whilst the other 200 ate Microwave prepared food. Half an hour after the meal, the researchers took blood counts from all participants. The first group with the traditionally prepared food had a normal blood count. The second group (the people eating Microwave food) had a blood count similar to cancer patients!

Thawing food by microwave (even if only for a few seconds) destroys the nutrition. For those mothers who use a microwave oven to warm up their baby's bottle, they would do better to invest a little more time and use a more traditional way.

The US-authority for radiation protection (NCRP) published their research at the end of the eighties about the higher malformation in children from mothers using microwave ovens.

It often occurs that people exposed to this type of strain develop itchy skin, swollen legs, eye problems, allergies, hay fever and rashes, yet they have no idea where the complaint comes from. At the beginning they are likely to have swollen lachrymal sacs – usually indicated as kidney problems. It's not the fault of the kidneys that they are unable to detoxify, it is because of a clogged or sluggish metabolism.

Often upon arising people are more tired than in the evening when they go to bed. Some suffer from neck tension and pain in the cervical vertebra, migraine, eye problems and tingling arms.

Geopathic areas

It is a proven fact that there are: water veins, earth grids (Curry net, Hartmann grid), geological faults, and radioactive radiation. Their influence on our system is tremendous. People who sleep in a bedroom with radiation will suffer from insomnia, feel cold at night, have nightmares, night sweats, nervousness,

---

[3] *Journal of Natural Sciences*, 1998

depressions and many more serious complaints.

Watch your cats as they are radiation seekers, dogs however will never rest where there is radiation. This kind of phenomena also occurs in nature, as farmers will tell you that some animals like; ants, termites, owls, snakes and bees prefer to stay in places of radiation. However, some trees do not grow in radiation zones.

Be careful of where your children sleep because if they sleep in a radiation zone, they may toss and turn during sleep or have bed-wetting problem. These signs have to be taken seriously as they could indicate strong influences on the state of health. Many people, who had years of unsuccessful allopathic treatments, have recovered after their sleeping area was neutralized.[4]

Noxious Geopathic areas (Greek: GEOS = earth, PATHOS = suffering)

o   Waterlines: This ionized negative radiation is related to insomnia

o   Geologicle rupture: The tectonicale pressue from the shifting earth plates is related to backaches, joint pains as well as malfunctioning vital organs, headache and dizziness

o   The Earth magnetic field: Also known as the Hartmann Lines, where intersection points are related to various illnesses

o   Curry-line: The intersection point of the diagonal, reltes to organic inflammation due to too much energy or functional disorders as well as energy blockages due to too little energy flow in sleeping areas.

Amalgam fillings

Amalgam fillings used for dental work are one of the scourges of modern times and cause immense problems. In many countries Amalgam fillings are banned.

The FDA (US Food & Drug Administration) - www.fda.com advises the following:
Dental amalgams contain mercury, which may have neurotoxic effects on the nervous systems of developing children and fetuses.

Amalgam fillings are a mixture of 32 different metals. Some of them are highly toxic. A single amalgam filling with a surface area of only 1/2 square cm is estimated to release as much as 15 micrograms of mercury per day, primarily through evaporation and mechanical wear.

Dentists who apply amalgam fillings show overwhelming evidence of mercury poisoning. Autopsy reports of a group of dentists showed higher concentrations of the metal in their pituitary glands and double the number of brain tumours than among the ordinary population. More worrying, amalgam appears to cause subtle brain damage in dentists exposed to these types of fillings. Dentists only work with this material, we are the recipients of these toxins!

There is ample evidence of a relationship between amalgam and a number of diseases like Multiple Sclerosis, Alzheimer disease, fertility problems, hair loss, allergies and more.[5]

Through the combination of the different metals, saliva builds acidity. Some people are able to taste it. As part

of the saliva, the acidity reaches the stomach and colon. As saliva is usually slightly alkaline the acidity creates great strain. Chronic gastritis or diarrhoea or diverticulitis may occur.

Because of the metal in the mouth, an electrical charge flows with the following effects. As the teeth connect to the different parts of the body via the nerves, current caused by the amalgam fillings can disturb the normal

---

[4] *Geopathic Zones* – Luise Weidel, Germany 2000. Ancient knowledge and the latest scientific and medical findings.
[5] *What doctors don't tell you* – Lynne Mc Taggart, Glasgow 1996. The truth about the dangers of modern medicine

function of the nervous system. When this happens, the body develops complaints. For example; the triple tooth (eye-tooth) is related to the eye, the shoulder, kidneys, hips and the knee. Now it is possible that if your dentist inserts an amalgam filling into the eye-tooth, you could develop a pain in your shoulder. Obviously you don't know anything about the connection and think the pain is related to yesterday's heavy lifting. To sort this out, you go for therapy for an injured shoulder, but of course it does not improve. The pain is still there and you have spent a lot of money, just for the pleasure of a nice massage. However, if the filling falls out, the pain in your shoulder disappears.

Irrespective of what your dentist says, only use ceramic fillings. So far, these seem to cause no bodily dysfunction.

Another problem caused by this current is the disturbance of the flows in a large mass of nerves, which can cause migraine and allergies.

Poisoning from amalgam fillings can be a very slow process. Affected people often have loss of tonus (tissue quality below the skin covering) and the ability to take stress. They assume that their illness is because of age, genetics or job, while the real cause remains hidden.

If you are thinking of having amalgam fillings removed, choose a dentist who uses rubber dams and is meticulous in isolating the resultant debris. Afterwards it is advisable to do a detoxification (Chelation, Homoeopathy or Tissue Salts), which will help you to recover. This is the individuals' choice, but usually organisms need about a year to recover from amalgam filling poisoning. Because the release of poison from amalgam fillings is so toxic, it is advisable to not remove too many fillings at any one time.

Unfortunately there are other sources of mercury poisoning to our system, such as from vaccinations, as they are stored in mercury. Allopathic practitioners recommend that babies be vaccinated some 18 times before reaching the age of two years! No wonder children are ill and have lots of allergies.

Nutrition

There are many books on nutrition, diets and eating habits – all of which should help you. However, your emotional makeup influences not only the gastric juices in the body, starting from the saliva to the composition of the stomach acidity, but also how you absorb nutrition. Often the organisms of a person will not be able to take nutrition from the food, as the acidity of the fluids will prevent it.

Of course it is advisable to eat health giving food, with lots of vegetables and salads. These are fresh living foods, promoting vitality, cleansing the system and if organic, deposit minerals in the body.

Tissue Salts

If you should disregard the above advice, don't be surprised when you suffer from ill health or lack of energy. Problems first start to manifest on the physical level as a result of mineral deficiencies.

Tissue Salts are responsible for the proper course of cell function. If they are not sufficiently available, the organisms have to reduce this function to a minimum. Sometimes the deficiencies are so pronounced, that single processes in the body are no longer possible.
Tissue Salts have to be replenished, which is not always easy as there are other components involved to achieve holistic health![6]

There are pre-prepared Tissue Salt Combinations with an equal amount of all the main cell salts, which do help a person feel better. However, to facilitate the necessary balance it is recommended to take a personalized combination in order to reach optimal results.

---

[6] *Handbuch der Biochemie nach Dr. Schüßler* – Thomas Feichtinger, Stuttgart 1999

The Different Ways of Taking Tissue Salts

In principle, all Tissue Salts may be combined with any other salts and taken throughout the day. The absorbing of the active ingredients happens through the laryngeal mucous membranes of the mouth. The more urgently the body needs the Tissue Salts, the faster they dissolve or the sweeter they taste; this can also happen simultaneously. Taking more than one tablet at a time is a waste of the tablet. So the best results and most efficient way to get the minerals into your cells, is to take them one by one. The reason why it is important to take the Tissue Salts one at a time, is because of the size and the amount of the carrier (lactose) and its content of minerals. The given dose-size needs a certain amount of time to dissolve in your mouth, while the minerals are absorbed through the mucous membranes. Only a small quantity can be absorbed at a time. There are different possibilities:

1.   Separate your required daily tablets from the various bottles and put them into a dish or container and shake to mix. You can take this mixture at any time during the day, but only takeing one tablet at a time. Let it dissolve in your mouth.

2.   The minerals may also be dissolved in a bottle of still water. Take the solution in small sips. Retain each sip in the mouth for at least for 30 seconds.

3.   Diabetics and lactose intolerant people must dissolve the Tissue Salts. (48 tablets are equal to one bread unit.) In this case, first put water in a wide container, then carefully put the tablets in - don't stir. Let it stand for half an hour (or longer). The minerals should have dissolved by then. Pour this solution through a filter i.e., (coffee filter) as this strains out any lactose. The solution is now ready to take. Throw away the white lactose paste collected in the filter. Or if the solution is not filtered, sip some of the water into your mouth hold for 30 seconds and spit it out.

4   Schuessler's Tissue Salts may be given to babies: Dissolve the tablets and spoon feed the pulp to the baby. Another way is to bottle feed – but the effect is diminished.

5.   Animals will derive benefit when given Tissue Salts. Adapt the number of tablets to the size of the animal. Dogs like to lick the pulp of Tissue Salts from your hands, or you may dissolve the Tissue Salts in water and mix it in their food.

Tissue Salts are Compatible with other Treatments

Since Tissues Salts provide the organism with missing functional substances, they may be taken in conjunction with other medication, drugs, Homoeopathy, Acupuncture and Bach Flower Remedy etc. They will not conflict with other treatments, but rather support and promote them. For instance, in any remedy the organism is likely to react more favourably if the necessary mineral is available. In order to be able to do so, it needs to have enough available minerals for the necessary functional substances.

Combining Tissue Salts with Vitamins and Food Supplements

For complete health and well-being, you should try to achieve a balance between Tissue Salts, vitamins and food supplements. But remember your body is not able to absorb Vitamins, if you are short of minerals on a cellular level!

In Biochemistry the distinction between Vitamins and Tissue Salts are:
• Vitamins work outside of the cells – External cellular is called: Macro level
• Tissue Salts (minerals) work inside the cells – Intra cellular is called: Micro level

Missing minerals at the **Macro level** can't be supported with Dr Schuessler's Tissue Salts. This means if a person suffers from a deficiency on this level, it can't be improved by taking Dr Schuessler's Tissue Salts. They would have to change their lifestyle! Your M.D. can detect this kind of lack with a **blood count**.

Deficiencies at the **Micro level** are only detectable with **Facial Analysis**! When there is a shortage of Tissue Salts, it will show up as signs in the face or body. Fortunately these signs appear early enough for you to support the body with Tissue Salts before serious disturbances occurs. **To provide you with guidance for a daily face check, refer to the *A to Z guide* at the back of the book. These signs relate to the need of the different Tissue Salts.**

Your Body Talks to you, but are you listening?

Many people incorrectly assume that disease develops overnight, when in fact it takes many years. Disease is a loud scream for help. By taking Tissue Salts we don't suppress or fight against symptoms, we are working with the cause. And because of the clear Facial Signs we are able to support the cause directly. In the frenetic lifestyle that we find ourselves in, we don't listen to the signs that our body gives. Then when ill, we want to get well as quickly as possible, usually by taking suppressing drugs.

Would you do this with your car? You drive and suddenly there is a flashing red light. You go to a workshop and have them see to it. Once fixed, you drive back home. Next day you start the engine and drive to work. After a few minutes you hear a strange noise. Upon inspection, you find a loose screw and throw it away. Later on your car breaks down. Of course you wouldn't do that! You would seek the cause and repair your car.

If you carefully listen to your body, you will hear and feel its needs and would acknowledge the red light flashing. Be grateful if it is still flashing, some people's lights don't flash anymore! End of the story!

Significance of Nutrition and Hydration

There is an old saying; "If we eat incorrectly, no doctor can cure us – if we eat correctly, no doctor is needed". The saying still applies today. For health's sake it is advisable to buy organic food and try to avoid wheat, gluten and meat.

There is absolutely no way to achieve a constant state of wellness and an absence of illness without good nutrition. All living, rejuvenating, healing processes are intimately related to the work of nutrients. Not only do we need balanced nutrition to support our body, but also enough hydration for the eliminating of waste. The cells play a vital part and will not be able to function to capacity if the body is de-hydrated. The best way to hydrate the cells is with pure water and herbal teas.

Our body needs at least double the amount of fluids (water) to digest coffee or black tea. If you drink one cup of coffee you would have to drink a cup of water only to equalize the amount of fluid in the body. The Ayurvedic philosophy recommends drinking boiled hot water; it is normally easier to store in the body.

It is good marketing of the producers, as to why people start replacing water with sweet drinks, like Cola. These dehydrate and acidify the body and is pure carbon dioxide! In order to **neutralize 1 glass of Cola, it takes 32 glasses of high pH alkaline water!** Diet drinks are really bad for you. They may be lower in calories, but are high in sodium, which causes high blood pressure.

There was a competition at the Delhi University as to who could drink the most Coke? The winner drank 8 bottles and died on the spot! This was because there was too much carbon dioxide in the blood and not enough oxygen. From then on, the principal banned all soft drinks from the university canteen. It would be absolutely fantastic if this event were better known, simply to protect our children from these poisoning drinks.

We shouldn't forget that the effect of these types of beverages cause bone deterioration, kidney stones, diabetes, heart disease, cancer, tooth decay, back problems and other illnesses.

It is a well-known fact that high phosphorus and phosphoric acid, (these are found in meat and soft drinks) reduces calcium from the bone structures (bones, teeth and nails). The nutrition of today; consisting of lots of meat and soft drinks can also cause bone malformation in the foetuses of pregnant women. Not only loss of Calcium in the bone structure occurs, it also produces acidity in the body. This can cause gout, arthritis, allergies, tiredness, weak skin and more.

By the refining and processing of food, extracting and adding salts, sugars, chemicals, preservatives and colorants, the leftover natural minerals are destroyed. Aggravating this is the depleted minerals in fruit and vegetables, as a result of modern agricultural methods.

If we were cannibals, human meat is likely to be banned because the average body is so contaminated from; pesticides, artificial ingredients, toxic waste and drugs that we knowingly and unknowingly ingest. [7]

The above shows only part of the disaster of our nutritional consumption. Hopefully the message is strong enough to start a change in nutrition. Don't change everything in one day, rather establish a habit of making small daily improvements. For more information about nutrition and the effect on our body (mind & soul), read the relevant books.

Expectation of reactions

When disturbances in our organism interfere with our normal lifestyle, we use painkillers or antibiotics. In fact, not only are antibiotics bad for you, they only treat the symptoms. By using these unnatural agents other problems occur, such as the prevention of secretion of toxins and pathological substances and the inability of the body to create anti-bodies.

Any illness, not given a chance to heal properly, is re-circulated back into the body. Initially, the body copes, but lacks strength. This is evident by the weeks of exhaustion experienced after taking serious drugs.

Suppressing an illness, results in the body finding other ways to give you the message that all is not well. With the detoxification mechanism not functioning properly, nothing can be secreted. This will continue until the lifestyle has changed with improved nutrition or the source of the illness is treated.

Often people show reactions when they first take Schuessler's Tissue Salts. The same symptoms (not the illness) may appear from an illness of the past. These symptoms mean that the Tissue Salts are working and removing toxins from the body. As a result, people mistakenly blame Tissue Salts, thinking that they are allergic to them! As Tissue Salts are natural to the body, it is impossible to be allergic to them. However, there might be reactions from taking them.

Other steps to improve your health may include changing the position of the bed, removing TV, mirrors and cables out of the bedroom, working through mental blockages or other interventions.

The organism will maintain life as long as possible under any circumstances. However, the strains and stresses of modern lifestyle prevent us from having adequate vitality and concessions need to be made. The restrictions enforced by the body are made according to its own wisdom. They are enforced with the aim that life will be maintained as long as possible. Thus hair, nails, teeth or bones are no longer well supplied – due to deficiencies - or damaged cells that are not regenerated. They remain depleted because the body does not have enough working agents (minerals in the cell) to tackle the problem.

Why do we suffer from Allergies?

The body is overloaded as a result of the many toxic substances in the food we eat and the air we breathe. Toxic substances need to be removed from the blood, lymph's and liquid in the tissue, as well as the cell. The toxins gradually settle inside the cells where they damage the immune system. When the body is filled with toxic, pathological and stressful substances, we experience allergic symptoms from: medication, detergents, animal hair and many more. The body will over-react to even the smallest amounts of allergic foods, causing impeded mobility or chronic disease.

If the bedroom has electrical pollution, the build-up of toxins and stressful substances is even more pronounced. Organisms are unable to carry out the necessary detoxification.

---

[7] *The Hundred-Year Lie* – Randall Fitzgerald, 2006. How food and medicine are destroying your health

Vital Need for Detoxification

One of the most intense secretive processes to get rid of the toxins, is achieved by sweating. There are two different forms; active and passive sweating.

Active sweating occurs during concentrated physical exercise and helps organisms to secrete harmful substances, collected in the subcutaneous area.

Passive sweating also helps to eliminate harmful substances. This may take place in a sauna or in a bath. If you prefer a bath, your body will start to sweat after around 30 minutes and secrete harmful substances as long as you keep the temperature constant slightly above 37 °C.

Toxic substances accumulate at night in the mucous membranes of your mouth. It is important to clean your teeth, wash out your mouth and gargle in the morning before you drink or eat anything. If you don't, you will swallow the accumulated toxins and distribute them throughout the body.

Recommended Prevention

Neither the years of depletion, nor the impact of stress on our bodies should be underestimated. After the symptoms have disappeared, it is essential that the bodies own deposits are replenished. These are the buffers for times of stress. When stress occurs, the body can access the deposits. Such is the need for the deposits that even a remotely satisfactory prophylactic regimen needs to deal with the replenishment of the mineral deposits in the body to build resistance. This may take weeks, months or even years, depending on the severity of the depletion, and particularly if a person has burnout due to repetitive high stress loads.

A high stress life style uses up the functional substances, so to prevent breakdown Tissue Salts should be taken. By doing so, the body will not need to fall back on its reserves. If the constant need is not replenished, ailments will ultimately occur. Eventually, these will need to be tackled, otherwise a chronic illness will develop. Once this happens, it will not be so easy to treat.

Even if there are no medical complaints, Tissue Salts should be used as a preventative. They will also reverse and delay the ageing process.

In order to support a faster recovery from infectious disease or simply keeping the mineral level in the cells constant, take the following daily mixture to boost your immune system.

	Immune system booster	
No 4 - Ferr phos.	Activates the power of resistance, Antioxidant	15 tabl/day
No 6 - Kali phos.	Energy regeneration together with No 9	10 tab /day
No 9 - Nat mur.	Regeneration, restoration of fluids	10 tab /day
No 21 - Zinc mur.	Tonic for immune system	15 tab /day
No 26 - Selenium	Regulates the joining together of cells and Boosts the production of antibodies Hinders the virus multiplying, Anti-inflammatory	15 tab /day

If you take this mixture regularly (especially during the season of colds and flu) you may resist infections.

After cure: Once you have cleaned your body from all the toxins and refilled all the empty deposits, support your body with mineral with the following; numbers 1 to 12 each between 1 and 3 tablets daily.

The ingenious body system

If the mineral deposits decrease as a result of high demands, the body will not react immediately with a breakdown. The human body is very clever as it collects deposits of all the required materials, enabling it to react immediately when strain occurs. Short-term deposits, can be depleted as a result of a stress situation.

The consequence of the decreasing deposits will be a restriction of the body. If the deficiency is allowed to increase, less important parts of the body will suffer, such as; problems with hair and nails, wrinkles, tiredness or an unhealthy skin complexion. If the deficiency continues and no replenishing takes place, the body will no longer be able to take care of the important life functions!

This shows how important and vital it is to replenish the deficiencies whilst at an early stage. Therefore detection is vital and this is where Facial Analysis comes in!

Facial Signs related to deficiencies

Dr Schuessler detected that, not only does a lack of minerals disturb the body, but they are also reflected in the face. He found that Facial Analysis was a wonderful analytic tool to identify and to interpret deficiencies. Schuessler's followers, Dr Kurt Hickethier and Mrs W Sonner published a book called, *'Sonnerschau'* in 1936 on Facial Analysis.

Facial Analysis proved that every disease causes certain mineral deficiencies, which can be seen in the face and if left untreated may cause disease. As a result, Facial Analysis and the use of Tissue Salts has experienced a large growth in popularity. In fact, Facial Analysis and Tissue Salts have survived a century of medical advancement, mainly due to the fact that Tissue Salts work *with the cause* and not only with the symptom.

In the following pages you will learn the facial signs that reflect mineral deficiencies, as well as personality traits or compulsive behaviour.

N.B, The pictures used in this book are of clients. All were happy to be included (all have given their permission to use the pictures), as they have seen the results of the use of Tissue Salts and want others to derive the same benefit.

No 1 – Calcium fluoratum – Tissue Elasticity Restorer

Calcium Fluoride helps maintain tissue elasticity and is beneficial for conditions associated with over-relaxed fibres, general relaxation of the tissue, such as; piles, sluggish circulation and eczema. This includes dilated blood vessels with haemorrhoids, **enlarged** veins and varicose veins. The salts assists normal blood circulation and the treatment of cracked skin, muscle strain and injured ligaments. It may also be indicated with diseases affecting the surface of the bones, cuts in the skin and if the tooth enamel is in poor condition.

Deposit:
Calcium Fluoride is found in the enamel of teeth and bone surfaces.

Cause of deficiency, amplification:
Extreme variation in temperature, seasonal or at work (bakery, butchery and the like), during the cold season especially if outside. The superficial muscles and vessels contracts to avoid heat-loss. In the warmth (inside) they stretch out again, causing cracked skin, consuming a lot of thisTissue salt!

Reactions:
Pain in joints, indicates the missing function agent, the symptoms are exaggerated in the body.

Facial Signs:
• Brownish–blackish discolouring
• If very deficient, a furrow under each eye
• Bluish and often cracked lips
• Transparent teeth-tips, Dental problems like caries
• Flabby skin

Body Signs:
• Broken skin, cracked heels
• Calluses and hard skin on hands, feet and elbows
• Stretch marks
• Spastic colon
• Varicose veins
• Feet problems (flatfoot, splayfoot, twisted ankles)

Psychosomatics / Characteristic Signs:
- Fear of not being good enough
+ Confident

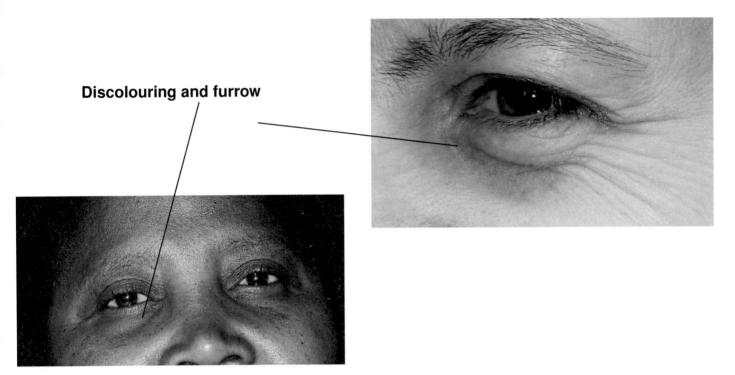

Discolouring and furrow

Brownish discolouring

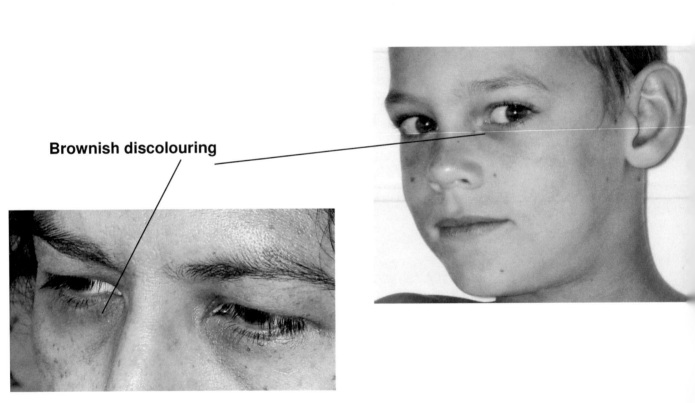

No 2 – Calcium phosphoricum - Cell Restorer

Calcium phosphoricum helps build the cells, as it splits protein into amino acids, these being the building blocks of all cell formation. It generates blood corpuscles and may assist during teething. It aids the prevention of muscular cramps and pain during menstruation and is especially helpful for young girls. It is beneficial for bone diseases, constitutional weakness and ailments that prove obstinate. Calcium phosphoricum is a general nutrition tonic and often indicates that there has been defective nutrition. As this Tissue Salt assists in digestion and assimilation it is excellent after surgery when the digestive system has slowed down. Calcium phosphoricum is recommended for the treatment of anaemia in conjunction with Ferrum phosphoricum.

Deposit:
Calcium phosphate is found in the inside of bones and teeth, muscles, blood.

Cause of deficiency, amplification:
Cold feeling; tensed muscles need lots of energy, causing feelings of coldness. There may also be the grinding of teeth.

Cravings for or refusing of: Bacon, ham, Ketch-up, mustard, smoked meat and milk.

Reactions:
Painful reactions when cramped muscles loosen up.

Facial Signs;
• Pale transparent waxy-like looking skin
• Transparent teeth-tips
• White spots on teeth or nails

Body Signs:
• Allergies of protein, Gout attack
• Cramp in the calf
• Neck and shoulder pain, numbness, tingling hands and feet
• Osteoporosis
• Sleeping disorders
• Screaming small children, bed-wetting
• Blood disorders
• Obesity

Psychosomatics / Characteristic Signs:
- Fear of being being ignored, frightened, worried, introvert, shy
+ Confident

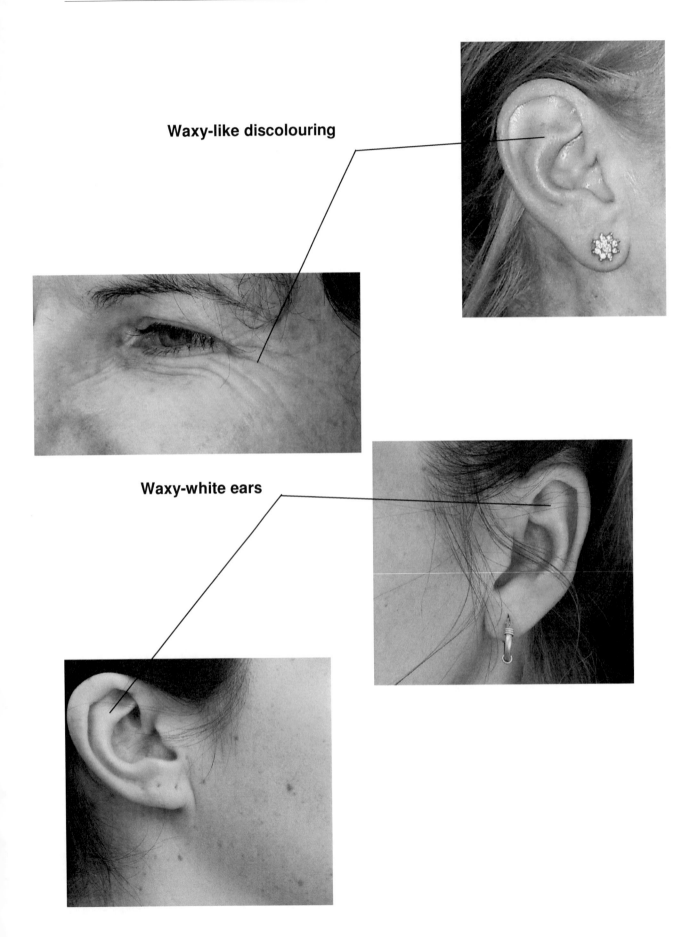

Waxy-like discolouring

Waxy-white ears

No 3 – Calcium sulfuricum - Blood Purifier, Purulent Agent

Calcium sulfuricum is a constituent of connective tissue, mucous membranes and skin. It helps clear away accumulations of non-functional decaying matter. This material may otherwise lay dormant or decay slowly whilst damaging surrounding tissue. Calcium sulfuricum is beneficial for slow wound healing, during the last stage of suppuration, for pimples, boils, carbuncles, ulcers, abscesses, etc. Calcium sulfuricum helps in the removal of waste products and has a cleansing and purifying effect throughout the system. This Tissue Salt supplements the action of Kalium muriaticum in the treatment of (adult) acne and catarrh and is an indicats if there is a deficiency in the connective tissues, where skin eruptions turn to abscesses and ulcers.

Deposit:
Calcium sulfuricum is found in bones.

Cause of deficiency, amplification:
Acidosis

Reactions:
None

Facial Signs:
• Alabaster white discolouring, like plasters
• Adult acne
• Boils, carbuncles, abscesses
• Thick wrinkles – so called compacted wrinkles (connective tissue).

Body Signs:
• Prolonged process of suppuration (pus)
• Gout, rheumatic complaints
• Gingivitis
• Bronchitis
• Epigastric discomfort

Psychosomatics / Characteristic Signs:
- To be open to everything might be an excessive demand; to be closed to everything would be an encapsulation
+ Cut off your nose to spite your face

Impure skin, adult acne

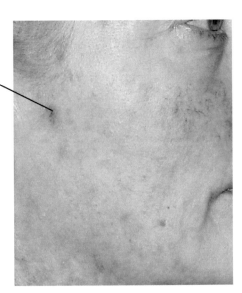

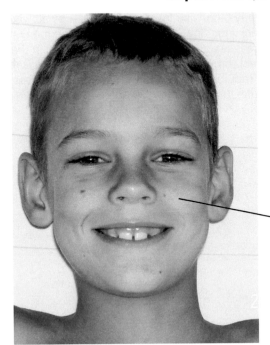

Shiny white skin

Entire white face

Impure skin, adult acne

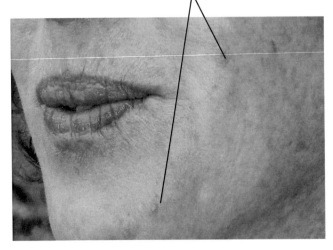

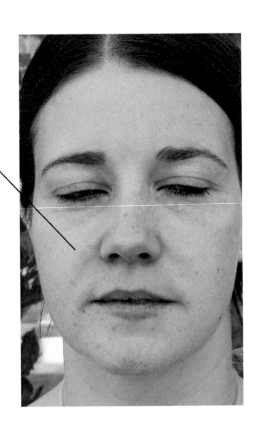

No 4 – Ferrum phosphoricum - Anti-Inflammatory

Regarded as the Oxygen Carrier, Ferrum phosphoricum is beneficial for any inflammatory or feverish condition. It is the chief remedy in headaches of children. Helps ailments arising from disturbed circulation – heat, pains, redness, throbbing, or quickened pulse. It is beneficial during the first stage of acute diseases, common cold, bronchitis, measles, respiratory infection, acute rheumatism, etc. This mineral assists in maintaining normal body resistance to disease. It may also be applied as a paste after being dissolved, on wounds, cuts and abrasions where there is bleeding (the carrier lactose acts as an antiseptic).

Deposit:
Ferrum phosphoricum is found in the root of the nose.

Cause of deficiency, amplification:
Coffee, black tea and cocoa (Theobromin!) use lots of FP.

Reactions:
In the early stages, a slight increase of the signs of illness is possible.

Facial Signs:
• A bluish-blackish shadow or a colourless furrow at the bridge of the nose
• If very deficient, dark circles under the eyes
• Hot red ears
• Warm-reddish flushed face (cheeks, forehead)
• Inflamed skin spots, impurity
• Inflamed eyes, red with burning sensation

Body Signs:
• Tiredness, exhaustion (lack of oxygen in the blood)
• Shortness of breathe
• Sun intolerance
• Weak concentration
• Low resistance
• Flu and colds
• Headache (behind eyes)
• Menstruation complaints

Psychosomatics / Characteristic Signs:
- Friction with the inner and outer world
+ Consent to the flow of life

Discolouring and furrow

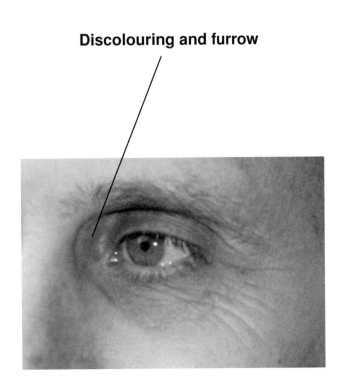

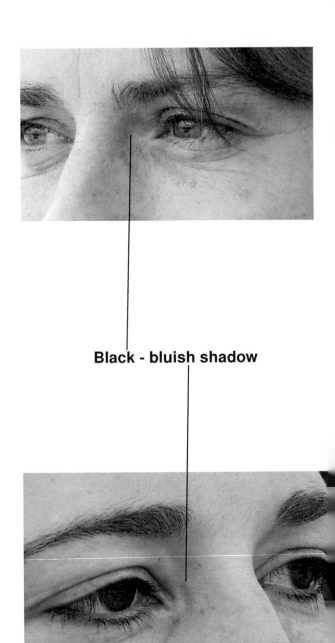

Black - bluish shadow

Black – bluish discolouring

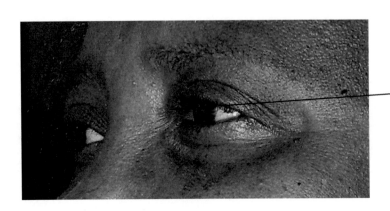

No 5 – Kalium muriaticum - Detoxifying Agent

Kalium muriaticum is helpful for conditions affecting the respiratory system - colds, coughs, bronchitis, tonsillitis, as well as ulcerated sore throat, catarrhal infection of the middle ear. It also aids the reduction of mucus congestion, curing colds and sinusitis. Kalium muriaticum is beneficial for the lymphatic glands and in problems associated with thick white or greyish discharges, or where there are glandular or chronic rheumatic swellings. Works well with Calcium sulfuricum to cleanse and purify the blood. It is useful in infantile eczema, and with Ferrum phosphoricum for a variety of children's ailments. Other key symptoms include white-coated tongue and light coloured stool. Kalium muriaticum is important in digestive disturbances, especially from eating fatty or rich food.

Deposit:
Kalium muriaticum is found in the bronchial tube, mucous membranes and glands.

Cause of deficiency, amplification:
The body needs a lot of this mineral to deal with alcohol, dairy products as well as electro pollution.

Cravings for or refusing of: Marzipan

Reactions:
Fast reaction, for a while an increase of the symptoms is possible.

Facial Signs:
• A milky-reddish/purple to milky-bluish area around eyes, mouth or entire face
• Bluish eyeballs
• Spider-veins
• Red eye blood vessels
• Grutum (small hard white spots)

Body Signs:
• Glandular complaints
• Nausea – morning sickness in pregnancy
• Cough with white mucous

Psychosomatics / Characteristic Signs:
- Overemotional
+ Appropriate emotions

Bluish eye-balls

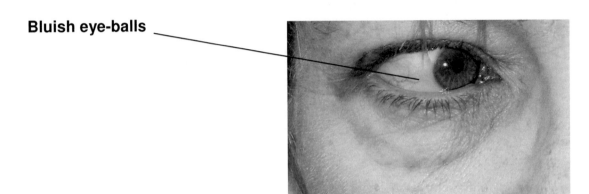

Spider vessels

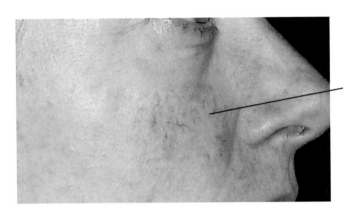

Milky-bluish-reddish discolouring

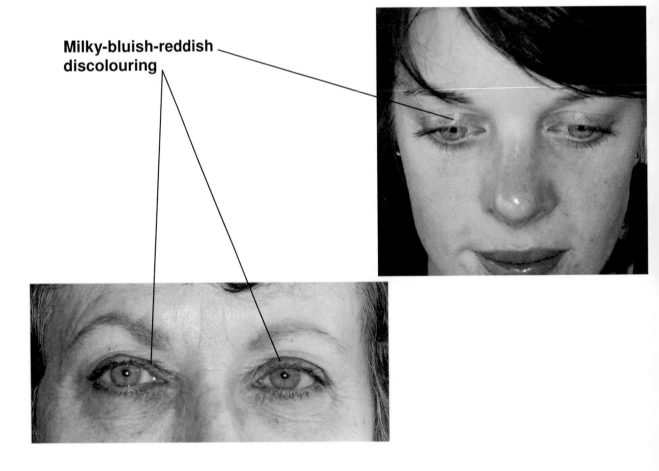

No 6 – Kalium phosphoricum - Nerve and Brain Cell Agent

Kalium phosphoricum is useful for the treatment of nervous conditions such as headaches, nervous exhaustion, dyspepsia, insomnia, depression and lowered vitality. Also use for shingles and nervous asthma together with Magnesium phosphoricum. It is particularly valuable for emotional irritability, depression, nervousness, and children's tantrums.

Deposit:
Kalium phosphoricum is found in temples, spleen and nerves.

Cause of deficiency, amplification:
It is advisable to check the bedroom for radiation. A deficiency of this mineral is usually related to a strain during sleeping time. Recommended before, during and after any special effort, to replenish deposits.

Cravings for or refusing of: Nuts

Reactions:
For fever it can be also be useful to give Calcium phosphoricum

Facial Signs:
• Greyish undertone around mouth and chin or entire face
• Dull eyes
• Sunken and greyish temples

Body Signs:
• Foul breathe
• Physical exhaustion
• Agoraphobia
• Gingival bleeding, recession
• Despondency, moaning

Psychosomatics / Characteristic Signs:
- Feels demands are excessive. Things are never good enough.
+ Performs to rhythm between tension and relaxation - action and retreat

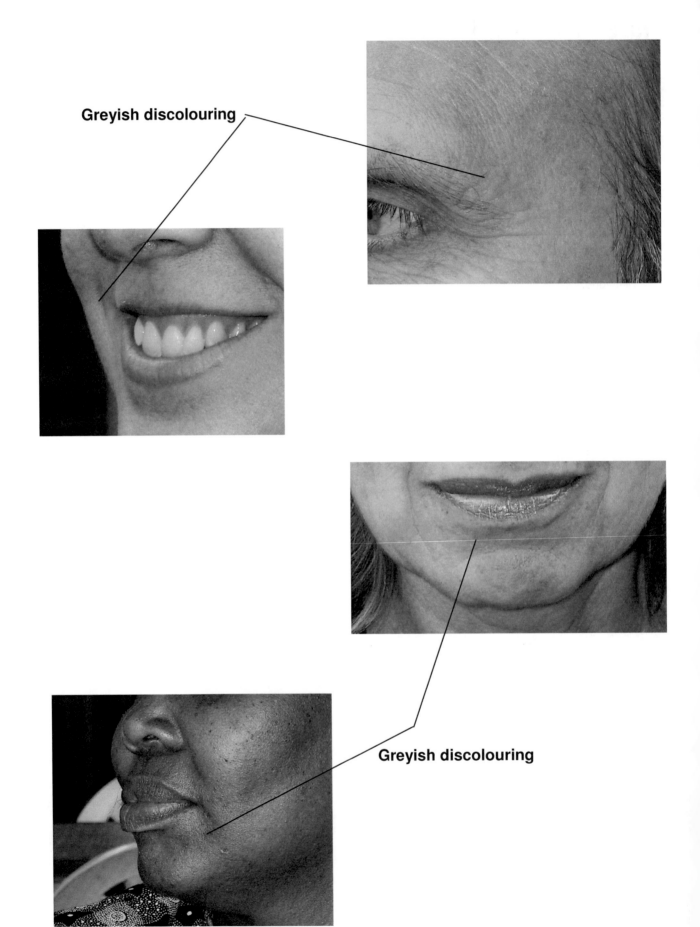

Greyish discolouring

Greyish discolouring

No 7 – Kalium sulfuricum – Metabolism, Pancreas Conditioner

Kalium sulfuricum works in conjunction with Ferrum phosphoricum as an oxygen carrier where together they have a beneficial effect on respiratory and circulatory functions. Kalium sulfuricum is also useful for skin complaints and minor eruptions such as scaling or sticky exudation as with dandruff, chicken pox, etc. Kalium sulfuricum may also give relief from catarrhal problems associated with yellowish or greenish discharge (mucous membranes of the nose or vagina). A deficiency of Kalium sulfuricum causes a lack of oxygen leading to instances of coldness, heat and shifting pains in the limbs. It is valuable in the treatment of Psoriasis, Athlete's foot and brittle nails.

Use towards the end of a cold, when discharge is profuse and frequent. It is sometimes beneficial for shifting acute rheumatic pains. It opens the pores of the skin, brings blood to the surface and promotes perspiration. As a result it is often beneficial in alternation with Ferrum phosphoricum for fever, when the temperature rises in the evening.

Deposit:
Kalium sulfuricum is found in the pancreas.

Cause of deficiency, amplification:
People taking a thyroid remedy usually have a need for oxigen; the remedy seems to put a strain on the liver and pancreas. To resolve this, large doses of Kalium sulfuricum are required.

Reactions:
Kalium sulfuricum dissolves the waste; to transport it out of the body, you will need Natrium sulfuricum (in a higher dosage) otherwise you will get toxic symptoms (waste jam).

Facial Signs:
• Brownish-yellow discolouring around chin and eyes or entire face
• Pigmentation complaints
• Ageing spots

Body Signs:
• Need for fresh air
• Naevus (birthmarks)
• Diabetes – high blood sugar
• Epigastric complaints, feeling of fullness

Psychosomatics / Characteristic Signs:
- Anger, self-denial, slavishly fulfilment of expectations
+ Strong opinions, feelings, protests, objections and demands on life

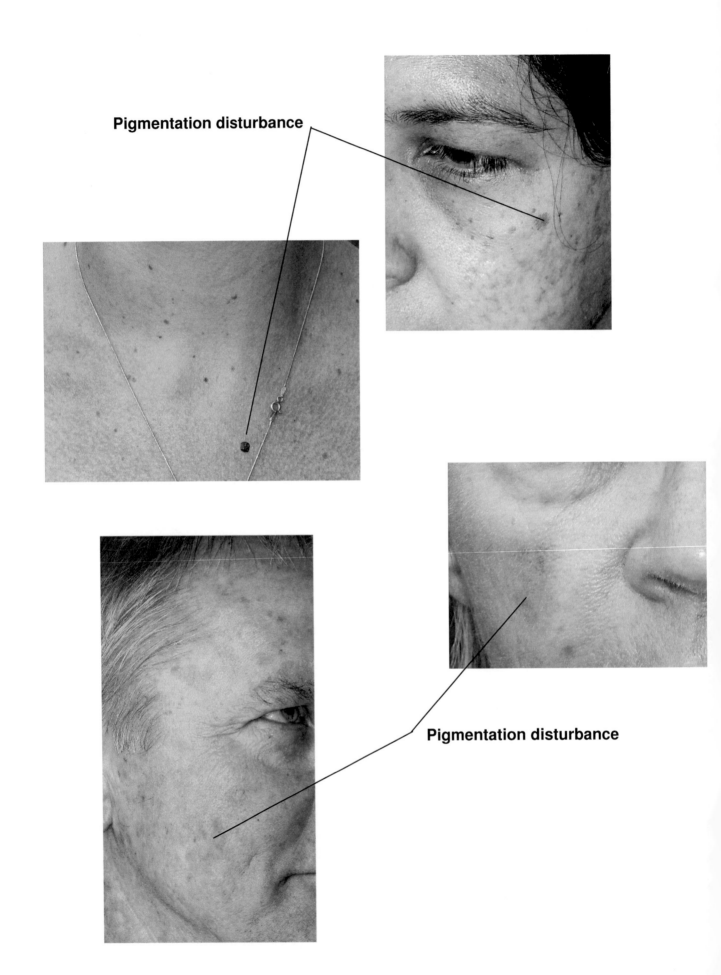

Pigmentation disturbance

Pigmentation disturbance

No 8 – Magnesium phosphoricum - Pain-and Cramp-Killer

Another mineral element of bones, teeth, brain, nerves, blood and muscle cells. Magnesium phosphoricum is beneficial for the treatment of muscular cramps, spasms and minor nerve problems. It is the main remedy for complaints of a spasmodic nature, such as colic, menstruation cramps, palpitations, spasmodic cough, toothache, neuralgia and acute pains in general. It is an important remedy for baby's colic, as it's beneficial in many cases of exhaustion due to emotional upset.

This salt quickly relieves muscular twitches, hiccups and sharp twinges of pain. Symptoms are usually worse when it is cold (better when it is warmer), pressure or bending over. Take frequently until relief is obtained.

Deposit:
Magnesium phosphoricum is found in nerves, heart, and glands.
Cause of deficiency, amplification:
Electromagnetic strain consumes a lot of Magnesium phosphoricum

Cravings for or refusing of: Alcohol, chocolate, coffee, and nicotine.

Reactions:
Fast results as a 'Hot 8'; dissolve 7-10 tablets Magnesium phosphoricum in half a cup of boiled water. Take as hot as possible, sip often, and retain it in the mouth (30 seconds), before swallowing. Helps with headaches and improves sleep.

Facial Signs:
• Pinkish to crimson spots beside nasal wings
• Face can be flushed
• Vibrant crimson spots
• Frantic blush
• Red flush after a meal or drinking alcohol

Body Signs:
• Menstrual pain
• Migraine
• Constipation
• Irregular pulse
• Stage freight

Psychosomatics / Characteristic Signs:
- High tension due to fear of disgrace and inferiority
+ Trust in oneself, confidence and strength of character

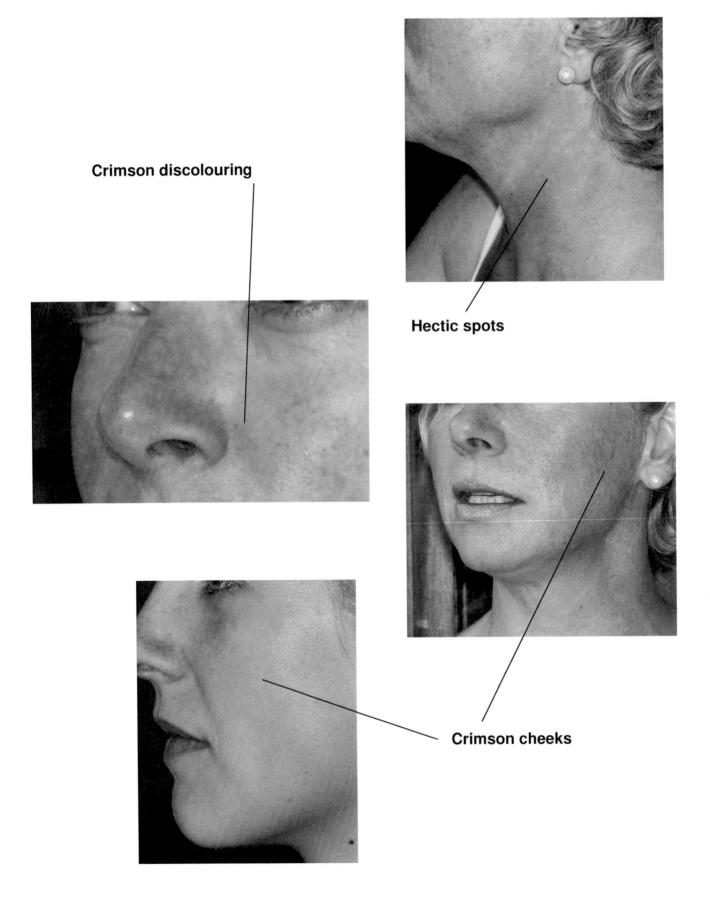

Crimson discolouring

Hectic spots

Crimson cheeks

No 9 – Natrium muriaticum - Water Distributor

Excessive moisture or dryness throughout the body is a good indicator for Natrium muriaticum, the symptoms can be many and varied. One of the most important Tissue Salts, as two thirds of our body is made up of water and hence dysfunction in this area can lead to widespread problems. Considered the Water Salt, Natrium muriaticum helps control the degree of moisture in the tissues, and as such is beneficial for temporary relief of conditions such as watery colds, (runny nose and eye watering symptoms), sneezing, un-refreshing sleep, low spirits with a hopeless feeling, loss of taste and smell, dry skin, headache with constipation.

Deposit:
Natrium muriaticum is found in the mucous membranes.

Cause of deficiency, amplification:
Excessive use of salt, drinking more liquids than the body asks for. The body has to dilute lots of fluids, like coffee, soft drinks, beer and wine.

Cravings for, or refusing of salt and spicy food

Reactions:
Once a cartilage starts to heal, there can be pain from hardened and dry cartilages.

Facial Signs:
• Spongy and dry skin
• Extremely large pores
• Shine of gelatine on upper and under lid
• Dull eyes

Body Signs:
• Dandruff, dry skin
• Cracking joints
• Allergic Rhinitis, Sinusitis, Mucous membrane complaints
• Cold hands and feet
• Burning pharynx (upper part)
• Excessive or no thirst
• Craving for salty food
• High or low blood pressure

Psychosomatics / Characteristic Signs:
- Pouting, conceit, freezing, insulted
+ Trusts ability to find ways to approach other people

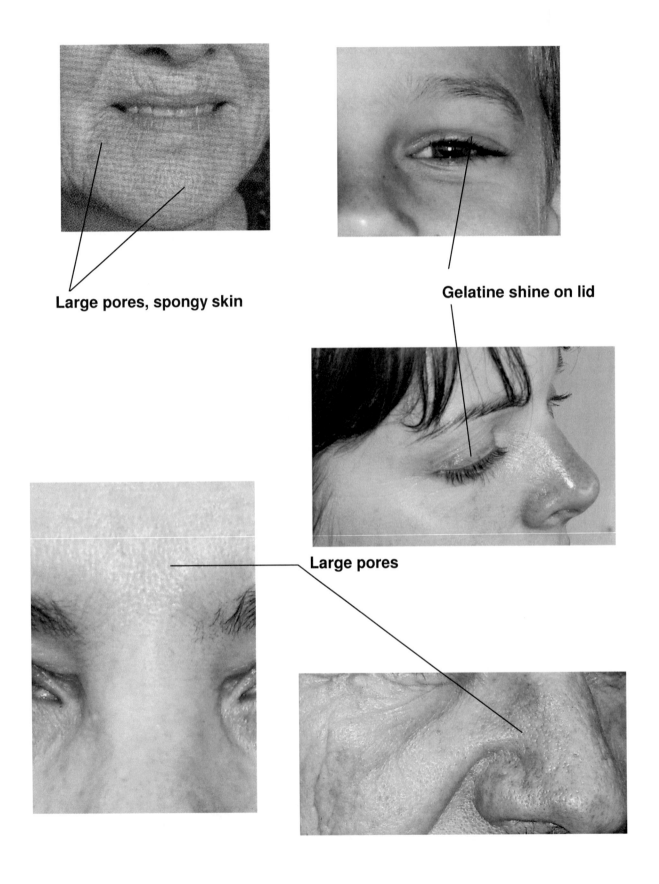

Large pores, spongy skin

Gelatine shine on lid

Large pores

No 10 – Natrium phosphoricum - Acidity Neutralizer

Natrium phosphoricum helps maintain the alkalinity of the blood, emulsifies fatty acids and keeps uric acid soluble in the blood. Thus, Natrium phosphoricum may also help young children who have been fed too much sugar and suffer from an acid condition. It also aids the temporary relief of gastric indigestion, dyspepsia, heartburn and intestinal worms.

A constituent of blood, muscle, nerve, brain cells and the fluid between cells. Natrium phosphoricum is needed with all complaints related to hyper-acidity. Also regulates bile. Use to treat gastric reflux or indigestion, all types of inflammation particularly relating to gout or rheumatism, burning with diarrhoea and stinging vaginal discharge.

Deposit:
Natrium phosphoricum is found in the Lymph's.

Cause of deficiency, amplification:
Nutrition has the most important effect on our acid metabolism. An increase of acidity due to sweets and soft drinks occurs.

Cravings for or refusing of; Sweets, desserts, butter

Reactions:
A short-term heartburn is possible, due to the fall-out of uric acid in the stomach. To improve the condition may require a few days.

Facial Signs:
• Blackheads and pimples
• Greasy / weak hair
• Greasy skin (T-bar)
• Acid wrinkles around the mouth
• Acid spots in the face
• Double chin
• Reddish chin (due to acidity)

Body Signs:
• Heartburn
• Swollen lymph's
• Craving for sweets
• Tiredness

Psychosomatics / Characteristic Signs:
– Pressure, violence (even to one's self), unreasonable effort, anxious, apprehensive
+ As much effort as necessary and no more, gentleness, sensitiveness

Pimples, impure skin

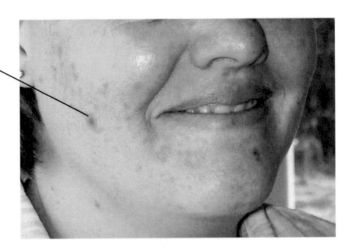

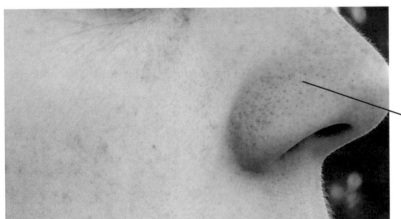

Blackheads

Greasy, weak hair

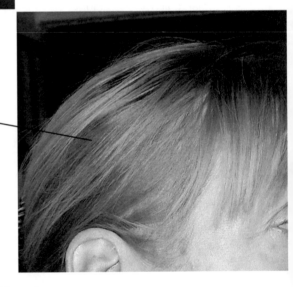

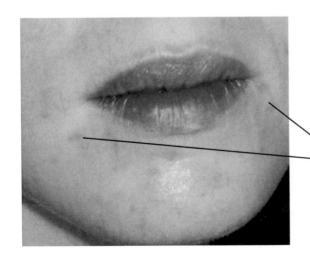

Pimples, acne

No 11 – Natrium sulfuricum - Liver Cleanser

Eliminates excessive water from tissues, blood and other body fluids. Acts as a cleanser and purifier of toxins from the fluid surrounding the cells in the body. It is necessary for the healthy functioning of the liver, spleen, kidneys and pancreas. Indicated for all ailments of or affecting the liver e.g. biliousness, liver troubles, digestive upsets and sandy deposits in urine, brown-green coating of the tongue, bitter taste. Particularly important in treating rheumatic complaints, gout and influenza as it eliminates the associated toxic fluids from the system. Helps dispel languid feelings experienced during humid weather.

Deposit:
Natrium sulfuricum is found in liver, gallbladder, and blood vessel walls.

Cause of deficiency, amplification:
Electromagnetic strain, alcohol, cigarettes and coffee.

Reactions:
Diarrhoea, pain in the limbs, itching, headache, badly smelling wind, loss of hair.

Facial Signs:
• Olive-greenish discolouring around eyes, mouth, chin or entire face
• Olive-greenish eyeballs
• A red-purple discolouring of the nose
• Swollen lachrymal sacs
• Puffy eyes

Body Signs:
• Swollen hands and feet (water retention)
• Itchy skin
• Warts
• Herpes
• Solar eczema
• Liver problems

Psychosomatics / Characteristic Signs:
- At the mercy of fate, anger, hate, irreconcilability
+ Reconciled with life and the own insufficiency, flexibility

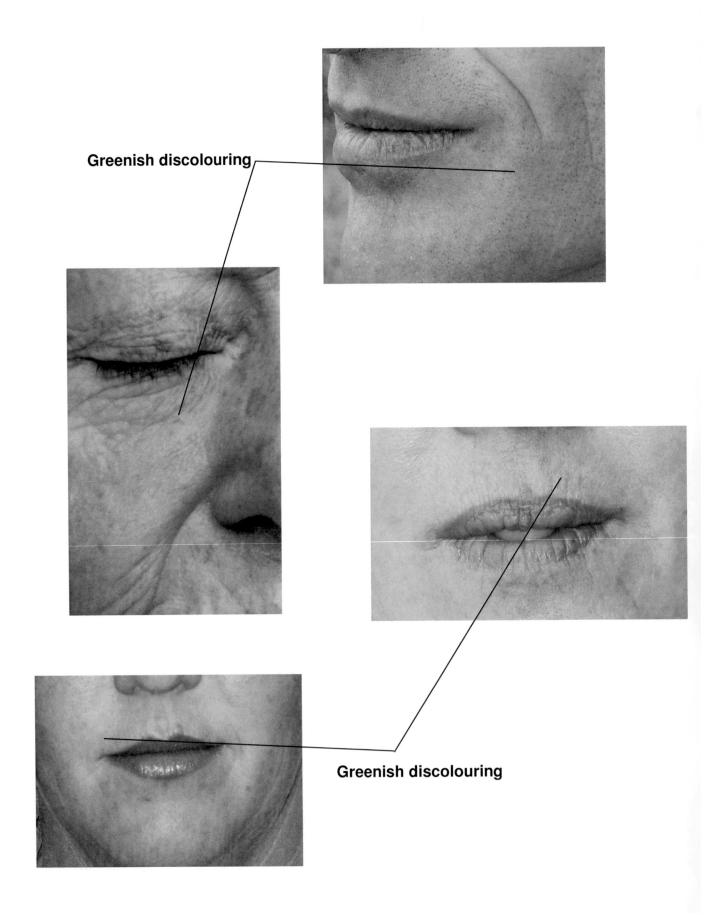

Greenish discolouring

Greenish discolouring

No 12 – Silicea - Skin and Connective Tissue Conditioner

A biochemical cleanser and eliminator, Silicea is part of all connective tissue cells. It promotes suppuration and the discharge of wastes, thereby often initiating the healing process by dispersing potentially harmful accumulates, such as skin eruptions and toxic blood conditions, abscesses, boils, etc. In the first stage of any swellings, Ferrum phosphoricum and Kalium muriaticum should be taken. If these tissue salts fail to eliminate the symptoms, Silica should be taken to ripen abscess and promote discharge. Silicea is beneficial for the health and strength of hair and nails. It helps eliminate foreign matter from the body and hence is helpful in the elimination of grass seeds. It complements Calcium, and in fact does the sculpting work to make sure that Calcium is laid down in the most appropriate areas (hence its role in Calcium deficiencies of the young and osteoarthritis of the old).

Deposit:
Silicea is found in the connective tissue, bones and skin.

Cause of deficiency, amplification:
Nerve-racking situations, stress, excessive need for harmony

Reactions:
Increased sweating (possibly with a bad smell), sweating hands, sweating feet.

Facial Signs:
• Wrinkling skin
• Shiny glossy nose tip or forehead (like a mirror)
• Hair problems
• Laughter-lines
• Compacted wrinkles
• When extreme the eyes may appear deeply sunken into their sockets

Body Signs:
• Nails with vertical lines
• Easily bruises
• Hypersensitivity to noise
• Hypersensitivity to light
• Easily sweating

Psychosomatics / Characteristic Signs:
- Feels guilty and responsible for everything, oversensitive, need for harmony
+ Learn to say NO!

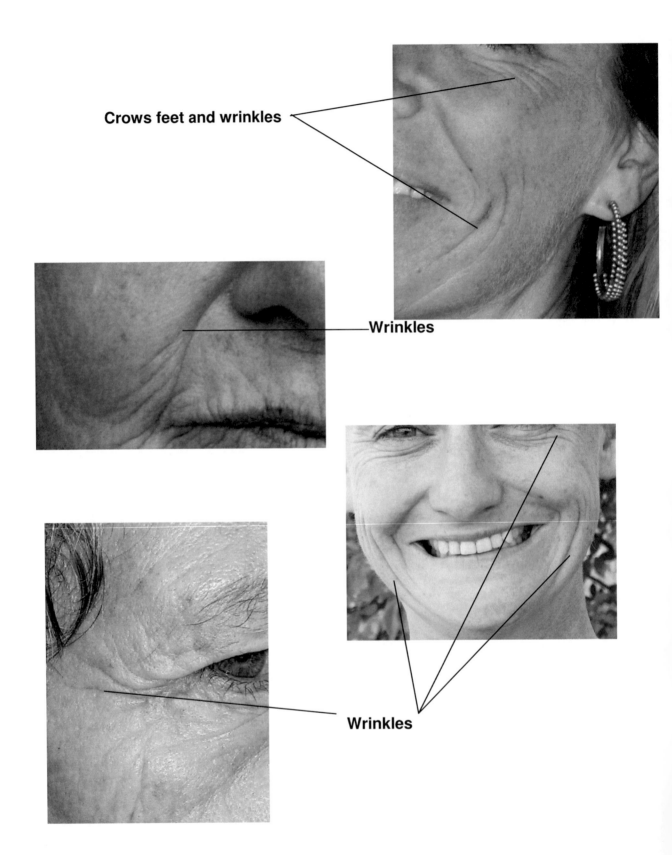

Crows feet and wrinkles

Wrinkles

Wrinkles

The 12 Tissue salts with functions & conditions

No	Tissue salt	Function	Organ/part of the body	Condition
No 1	Calcium fluoratum	Protection, elasticity, Tonus	Connective tissue (elasticity), bones, veins, skin, teeth, tendons, ligaments	Hard skin, cracked skin, varicose veins, ganglions, foot problems Osteoporosis
No 2	Calcium phosphoricum	Stability, protein process, reconstitute agent	Bones, muscles, teeth, spine, formation of blood	Osteoporosis, nose bleeding, formation of bones, teething, false posture, nasal polyp, heart hurry
No 3	Calcium sulfuricum	Purification	Liver, gallbladder, muscles (heart)	Chronic formation of pus
No 4	Ferrum phosphoricum	1st aid, oxygen Carrier	Blood, vessels, bowel	Concentration, low fever 38.8°), pulsating pain, inflammation
No 5	Kalium muriaticum	Function, detoxification	Glands, bronchus	Cough (whitish-mucous)
No 6	Kalium phosphoricum	Energy, tissue building	Spleen, nerves, muscles, psyche	Foul breathe
No 7	Kalium sulfuricum	Catabolism, oxygen transfer	Pancreas, liver, skin, mucous membranes	Need for fresh air, skin dandruffs
No 8	Magnesium phosphoricum	Drive, contraction	Heart, bowel	Need for chocolate, blush, stage fright
No 9	Natrium muriaticum	Detoxification, liquid/warmth regulator	Kidneys, blood, mucous membrane, cartilage	Cold (mucous watery-clear)
No 10	Natrium phosphoricum	Reduction of acidity, lipid metabolism	Stomach, tissue, lymph's	Pimples, blackheads, greasy/brittle hair/skin
No 11	Natrium sulfuricum	Catharsis, transportation	Liver, gallbladder	Swollen hands or feet, stinky winds
No 12	Silicea	Strength, connective tissue	Connective tissue (brittleness), skin, nerves, hair, nails	Sensitive to light, sciatic pain, groin hernia, sweating hands or feet

External application of Tissue Salts

After receiving a diagnosis of Facial Analysis, most people are keen to recuperate as quickly and easily as possible. To support this, the intake of Dr Schuessler's Tissue Salts can be taken externaly.

For *optimal absorption of minerals* (Tissue Salts taken through the skin), the water temperature has to be BELOW body temperature.

Full bath:

10 to 20 tablets of each of the recommended Tissue Salts for corresponding complaints dissolved in the water. Stay in the bath only for 8 to 10 minutes.

Foot bath:

5 to 10 tablets each of the recommended Tissue Salts (8 to 10 minutes). The foot bath can be extended up to the calf.

Underarm bath:

5 to 7 tablets each of the recommended Tissue Salts (8 to 10 minutes), can easily be done in the washbasin.

Hand bath:

5 to 7 tablets each of the recommended Tissue Salts (8 to 10 minutes). Use a basin or a small dish. Helpful, especially in cases of eczema and cracked hands.

Ablution:

If the person is not able to walk to the bathtub, then use a footbath. It is recommended to do ablutions by dissolving the recommended Tissue Salts in a washing bowl to wash the necessary parts of the body.

Coating:

The required Tissue Salts are made into a thick pulp with little water. A thick layer of the pulp is placed onto the injured skin. Cover with cling wrap, in order to keep the pulp humid. The carrier Lactose has an antiseptic effect. It is helpful to put this pulp directly on the wound.

First aid injuries:

Ferrum phosphoricum No 4 (relieves pain and stems blood flow)

Burns:

Lots of Natrium muriaticum No 9 and less Ferrum phosphoricum No 4

Additional Tissue Salts No 13 to 27

No 13 to 27 are supplementary substances. These have been discovered subsequent to Dr Schuessler research. They are well known in Europe and now available in South Africa. The additional Tissue Salts are very helpful and recommended for all modern illnesses.

No 13 – Kalium arsenicosum

Skin disorders
Helps: With itching eczema and states of weakness
Benefits: Menopause, intestinal complaints, warts

No 14 – Kalium bromatum

Nerve disorders and tension
Supports: Relaxation and sleep (tension related)
Benefits: Headache, migraine, restlessness

No 15 – Kalium jodatum

Anxiety and skin disorders, goitre
Helps: With depressed mood and dry skin
Benefits: Heart & brain activity, racing heart, dizziness, sweating

No 16 – Lithium chloratum

Blood cleanser
Helps: With conditions resulting from renal and urinary disorders
Benefits: Herpes, urethral inflammation, renal disease, arteriosclerosis

No 17 – Manganum sulfuricum

Cartilage & bone disorders
Helps: With rheumatoid arthritis, infertility, pregnancy, weak nerves
Benefits: Diabetes and hepatitis, osteoporosis

No 18 – Calcium sulfuratum

Blood cleanser
Promotes: Elimination of oxidation and harmful substances
Benefits: Exhaustion with weight loss, amalgam poisoning (Mercury)

No 19 – Cuprum arsenicosum

Central nervous system disorders
Promotes: Elimination of heavy metal poisoning, antioxidants
Associated: Parkinson, Multiple Sclerosis
Benefits: Articular pain, falling sickness, osteoporosis, pregnancy, rheumatism

No 20 – Kalium aluminium

Nerve disorders
Promotes:　　Elimination of heavy metal, helps nervous system
Associated:　Alzheimer, Parkinson
Benefits:　　Constipation, bloating, mucous membranes, dizziness

No 21 – Zincum chloratum

Blood disorders and acidity complaints
Promotes:　　Elimination of heavy metal and acidity
Associated:　Multiple Sclerosis
Benefits:　　Infertility, prostate complaints, white spots on nails, thin hair

No 22 – Calcium carbonicum

Bone and water imbalance
Helps:　　　With chronic mucous membrane complaints, severe exhaustion
Benefits:　　Anti ageing, permanent stress, weak constitution

No 23 – Natrium bicarbonicum

Acidity and waste
Boosts:　　　Metabolism, supports waste elimination
Benefits:　　Heartburn, uric acidity

No 24 – Arsenum jodatum

Allergies
Helps:　　　With symptoms of allergies, intestinal disorders
Benefits:　　Bluish extremities, bronchitis, hay fever, night sweat, rashes

No 25 – Aurum chloratum

Blood and liver support
Helps:　　　Wth women's diseases, hormone production and eye sight
Benefits:　　Blood pressure, liver disease, rheumatism, immune system

No 26 – Selenium

Immune booster
Supports:　　Immune system, heavy metal elimination and eye metabolism
Benefits:　　Dry skin, herpes, infertility, liver detoxification, psoriasis

No 27 – Kalium bichromicum

Sugar replacement
Support:　　　With diabetes and cholesterol
Benefits:　　Obesity, mucous membrane complaints, permanent stress

Psychic Phenomena in Biochemistry -
Individual structures of the various mineral substances

This expose is merely an introduction to the psychosomatic aspects of a lack of Tissue Salts. A detailed description of individual structures and their actions would fill an entire book.

As we all know, one of the most significant things in the life of a human being is the consequence of words and deeds experienced as a child. These experiences leave imprints on the personality for life.

It is unfortunate that many parents disregard the effects of their behaviour and words on their children. For example:
• children become injured on a physical and psychological level
• children do not react to injuries with anger; instead, they learn to love the pampering and the injury is quickly forgotten – yet the experience leaves its imprint in the cells
• the forgotten cell memory will re-surface later and cause, the now grown up person to release his or her anger on other, or through self-destructive behavioural-patterns, such as; smoking, drinking, drugs etc

What most people don't understand is that the consequences of such injuries, physical and psychological, also impairs the mineral balance, with the possibility of these mineral deficiencies becoming greater.

It is a well known that mineral deficiencies are transferred from mother to child during pregnancy. That's why an all encompassing Dr Schuessler's mineral supply is so vital during pregnancy. The correct mineral balance is important for the physical and psychological structure of the child. Either the child is born with a mineral deficiency (and the corresponding psychological defect), or vice versa. Subsequent dramatic life experiences will cause a mineral drainage and depletion, with very similar psychological results. And if the ensuing constrictive behaviour pattern is not changed, mineral deficiencies will deteriorate further. However, if Dr Schuessler's minerals are administered judiciously, in the correct selection and dosages, the mineral balance on a cellular level will be restored and the body, mind and soul connection will return to harmony.

It is important to remember that we cannot get the necessary minerals from our nutrients, as most of the planet's soil has been leeched and depleted. Vitamins and supplements cannot take their place because they are "alien", and not the bodies own material as Tissue Salts are. They are also too large to be absorbed into the cells. Dr Schuessler's minerals are the only source of body own minerals which, due to a natural miniaturisation process, can be directly administered and absorbed into the cells.

No 1 - Calcium fluoratum

Fear of not being good enough - the need to make a good impression.

This Tissue Salt is in charge of all the body's sheaths. It is responsible for the protection of health as well as activating when there is a hardening or solidification in the tissue of the body which is in need of dilation.

The lack of this particular Tissue Salt is revealed through the fundamental fears of Inadequacy, resulting in inferiority complexes. These stem from the forgotten cell memory that was mentioned earlier.

Negative comments during childhood like, 'You'll never make it!' conjure up fear, tension and oppression. The incapability of dealing with expectations of others will constantly evoke and trigger this fear syndrome.

The deficiency can also be detected by facial analysis in the form of dark shadows or rings under the eyes. It can be treated with large amounts of Calcium fluoratum.

Many people believe that good relationships *should* be maintained with all people that they come in contact with. The reality is that there is a need to make a good impression and boundaries are not set. The setting of boundaries is also closely related to the capability of saying, 'NO' when required.

The tension created by not being able to express an opinion or viewpoint, can lead to an obstinate negative behaviour, which will gradually cause a clogging up and stifling of all elasticity in the body. This in turn can lead to physical hypo-mobility, such as restricted movement and joint problems (osteoarthritis etc), and in extreme cases, can lead to physical symptoms such as hyper-mobility, i.e. joints and bones that become too mobile and can bend. This syndrome often manifest as an insecure posture.

A case in point - a father who forces his child to give away a favourite toy to another child may cause his child to experience a loss of protection, either for the toy or for himself. This could lead to psychological problems in adulthood; like having difficulties in relationships, or they may not be able to let go of people or possessions as time may dictate. They are generally in need of security and will insure themselves with many policies, not only for themselves but also their property as well.

The need to make a good impression on others can result in the 'freezing' of the person, by the stiffening of the body and facial expression. While the yearning of being accepted as a child will continue in adulthood, where a friendly face is given, whilst tears that are close to the surface. This results in a see-saw of extremes; frozen into inner stiffness - yet projecting maximum flexibility. People who rely on approval of others often feel that they have to earn the goodwill of others.

No 2 - Calcium phosphoricum

Fear of existence - provocation and determined to be noticed.

This Tissue Salt is essential for the health of the inner state and condition of the sheaths. It targets the tissue and liquids (e.g. blood) inside the protective sheaths. A person lacking this particular mineral is inclined to search for confirmation of his own existence. Being an impossible quest, he will develop latent existential fears, and thereby manages to alienate himself from natural acceptance of his own life. This may lead to provocation in order to get the desired reactions from fellow beings.

This particular mineral deficiency is also strongly connected to childhood experiences. All too often parents over-emphasise the importance of the child's cuteness, whilst also emphasising any awkwardness or clumsiness. The child soon learns that attention can be gained by acting in a certain way, thereby making it difficult for the child to relax into its own personality.

Psychologically, not to be heard or seen generates fear and produces the feeling of 'I don't exist'. Later in life, the body language and behaviour patterns demonstrate the, 'please forgive me for existing.' Whereas a child will focus all its attention on the outer world with the intention of confirming their existance.

Unfortunately, children of fear-inspiring parents are more prone to illness than those who were given support and freedom. A child that is constantly exposed to admonishment and restrictions cannot develop properly and will become rebellious at some stage. These young people will gravitate towards wearing flashy and conspicuous clothes and hairstyles, while their behaviour is overly loud and brash. They tend to be either obtrusive helpers, or display destructive tendencies in the quest to be noticed or seen. This behaviour causes tension in the body and is evident by a waxy paleness in the face, which is a clear sign of a Calcium phosphoricum deficiency. This is often accompanied by tension headaches as well as shoulder and neck strains.

As a result of perpetual muscle strains and the over-taxing the spinal column, bone growth and albumin development can become severely inhibited. This serious lack of care for the bone structure can also cause osteoporosis.

The search for recognition and acceptance causes the tendency to cling to another. This is because of the fear of being overlooked. There is also an aversion to entering confined spaces. Often, in a bid to be noticed, these maladies are clung to. This profile certainly does not allow for trust in life, or self-confidence.

No 3 - Calcium sulfuricum

Confusion, remains in a shell - fear of not being seen.

This person may have had some sort of shock, such as a breakup. Shocks always cause deficiencies of No 3 Calc sulf. As a result of the deficiency, the person is likely to go into a shell and withdraw from society. If the dificiency is not resolved the person is likely to become lonely and find it even harder to make friends.

Because these people crave acceptance and recognition by others, they lower their own expectations and desires. They do this while trying to meet the expectations of others, which usually results in failure. People in this condition also try to preserve their relationships at all costs. This demands great effort from them. But despite the clinging, a break of the connection can't be avoided. This break causes shock, despite all the effort made to keep the connection intact. The consequences of which may be to withdraw into a shell.

These people vacillate between extremes and rarely find balance. As a result the contraction of the superficial blood vessels leads to an extremely pallid countenance as an expression of the underlying mineral deficiency. The entire human tissue becomes condensed because of traumatic experiences, which can lead to fossilization of the person - character and body. Chronic suppuration, abscesses and furuncles are linked to this mineral deficiency as is bronchitis and chronic conditions such as gout, arthritis and skin diseases.

No 4 - Ferrum phosphoricum

Overheat - expects too much of oneself and others.

This Tissue Salt is connected to conflict situations and the associated friction. Friction can arise through changes in circumstances, or it can take the form of inner friction, stemming from expecting too much and a lack of self forgiveness.

Inner friction is evident in people who continuously rush and become impatient with those that do not have the same pace. They not only abuse themselves, they also abuse others by relentlessly perpetuating the unnatural pace. Being typically short tempered and tending to "overheat" for no serious reason.

This syndrome can easily cause higher "running temperatures" which uses up great amounts of Ferrum phosphoricum in the cells. However, a slow-paced person is subject to outside pressure because that person is not able to take his time. This may include the whole activity spectrum of reading, talking, moving, working, fighting etc. Adopting the pace of others will result in the individual being separated from his own truth. The feeling of not being recognised or seen is developed. This also causes a loss of **identity and the giving of personal power to another.**

Feeling overburdened, due to being exhausted makes it difficult or even impossible to produce or achieve. As a result, there is the thought that nobody cares. This vicious cycle consumes large quantities of Ferrum phosphoricum, with recognisable symptoms of reddened cheeks and hot ears.

Ferrum phosphoricum is also closely linked to the human development processes, as in conflict situations. Such situations will need working agents in the cells. Stable people do not expose themselves to conflicts, and therefore do not lack this mineral. Conflict situations use up large amounts of Ferrum phosphoricum in the body.

No 5 - Kalium muriaticum

Emotional - knowing how one should behave.

This Tissue Salt is associated with feelings and the quality of engagement with the world and life in general.

Kalium muriaticum is the substance and remedy of the glands and is an essential building stone of the mucous membranes situated in our sense organs. This demonstrates how this mineral is linked to feelings. Women for instance more readily display their feelings, while men tend to suppress them, as displaying feelings is considered a sign of weakness. Hence, both women and men can be diagnosed with a lack of Kalium muriaticum. Dr Schuessler's Tissue Salts will balance both extremes.

Our present state of mind is linked to how we are feeling. Too many influences and events in life distract us from our primal feeling of reality, thereby, often falling prey to the guidance or domination of other people.

Repression of feelings, or becoming alienated from them, leads to a harsh personality. It also leads to further problems and complications resulting in heart attacks and strokes. It is common knowledge that men are more prone to these and so this can be interpreted as a lack of sustenance for the heart.

Suppression of feelings in women leads to coldness, frigidity and problems such as Osteoporosis, which can be caused by the lack of bone care with cramping of the underlying musculature. The spine, as the 'back bone,' is the mirror of the personality; where courage for emotional involvement is lacking, the organism starts 'supporting' the weak spine with chronically tensed-up musculature. This severely stresses the vertebral discs. The sciatic nerve is usually the worst affected.

On a physiological level, the intensity of emotional activity quickens the depletion of Kalium muriaticum. If emotions are out of control, there is a possibility of an addiction or obsession. Take the example of a mother who claims, 'I always feel sick when my child is sick.' She attaches herself to the child's condition and may assert that this is love!

It is unfortunate that many parents stress the importance of possessions and status to their children, thereby creating emotional situations that heighten the depletion of Kalium muriaticum reserves.

Furthermore, this mineral deficiency may lead to physical contact phobias. A person with this complaint wants to scream and protest, but instead is nice and friendly, as that's how one is expected to behave.

No 6 - Kalium phosphoricum

Perfectionist and self-righteous - stickler of one's principles.

This Tissue Salt concerns itself with conflict intensity factors and (over) engagement in one's life. For the many life activities, we need energy, and we use Kali phos because it is in charge of the energy system.

The shortage of this Tissue Salt is evident when life has become too much to handle. The result of this will be the total depletion of energy. And if pushed too hard, can land the person in a world of despondency and demotivation, possibly even depression. In this situation, self-doubts will become the consequence of feeling overburdened by outside factors. This stands in direct juxtaposition to the internal overload situation. This reveals itself in moral judging of others in order to justify and bolster self-worth. 'I know what is right, and I have my principles', you'll hear him say. Such self-righteousness and lack of trust in others generates enormous tension and consumption of Kalium phosphoricum.

Excessive stress is also caused by trying to put certain ideals into practice, with failure being the likely outcome. People with this shortcoming lean towards perfectionism, sterility and excessive cleanliness in their homes. They expect too much from themselves and others. This fact is frequently mirrored in a face by a distinctly ashen complexion (i.e., doctors after difficult therapy sessions, or teachers after a class).

During childhood these people were often told to hang in there and bite the bullet, reacting with symptoms that often express themselves in the form of grinding teeth in an attempt to conquer and control the expectations of their world. This results in chronic gum bleeds right into adulthood. This problem cannot be solved by taking this mineral only, additional action is required.

Childhood experiences are also responsible for syndromes such as the need to comply with expectations, as well as the belief that one's behaviour and actions can determine and direct the wellbeing of another. Children often hear things like, 'I am really happy when you behave yourself', or 'Aren't we such a happy family when you do what we expect of you?' This type of childhood indoctrination demands self-confirmation from the outside, i.e. how good-looking you are? How incredibly well you performed some task? etc. Continued exposure to such expectation results in becoming a victim of self-doubt, followed by depression, which also mirrors linked physical symptoms. The depletion of this mineral results in conditions such as; despondency, tearfulness and dejection. This deficiency also causes halitosis, that ordinary brushing of teeth will not fix.

No 7 - Kalium sulfuricum

Self-denial - fulfilling the expectations of others.

This Tissue Salt is related to the fulfilment of expectations and demands, especially if the person finds these hard to comply with. It starts off with the distress caused by seemingly insignificant situations, as well as the desire to play an active role in life. Children are seriously stressed by not being recognised, especially due to a deliberate rejection at home.

Parents who do not show affection to a child (possibility as they are burdened by their own unresolved life issues), results in the child erecting a protective wall to block out the loneliness. In time this wall may become insurmountable, and figuratively speaking, the child will gasp for air because of a suffocating feeling. The increasing need for fresh air and freedom is due to a lack of this Tissue Salt. Therefore, this mineral is linked to asthma!

Such obsessive character structures demands an ever-escalating consumption of No 7 Kalium sulfuricum.

This mineral also governs the pigmentation substances of the skin, transports oxygen into the cells and rids them of stress substances, thereby cleansing the cells. If a deficiency is present, cells cannot be efficiently cleansed and will excrete toxins via the skin. This leads to itching and burning sensations that can develop into eczemas and even Neurodermatitis.

When a person feels shunned by others, he adapts in order to accept and comply with their demands and conditions, in the hope that they will finally recognise his existence.

Empowering and pleasing others requires a determined effort, while self concern increasingly falls by the wayside. The divergence between one's true feelings and one's actual behaviour becomes ever more pronounced. The need to scream and protest is replaced by good behaviour and friendliness.

Children are often told, 'I like it when you don't scream,' or 'I am really happy with you when you do what I tell you.' This prompts the child to do exactly what his parents tell him, without taking his own needs and feelings into consideration. The fact is, that this is a betrayal of the child's ego, generating anger and perhaps even hate. The feeling of wanting to give up on life and of being betrayed by others is common.

This inner contradiction exerts an enormous amount of stress on the pancreas, which consumes large amounts of Kalium sulfuricum. This situation can cause intense constrictions throughout the body and severely inhibits the breathing process. Oxygen should flood the cells but the constrictions prevent it from doing so. Molecular exchange activities become increasingly unfeasible, causing metabolic action to almost cease. Because the pancreas uses up large amounts of this mineral, its functionality is reduced, which can cause diabetes or metabolic disorders.

As self-denial is so prevalent with these people, they are attracted to regular use of the word, "one" in their speech, i.e. "one" can hide so effectively behind it. They also frequently say, 'The best thing for me is to be there for others,' or 'Can't you see how I sacrifice myself for you?' These are just a few typical examples of the kind of statements uttered by people with a pronounced lack of Kalium sulfuricum.

No 8 - Magnesium phosphoricum

The 'embarrassed' one. What will others think of me.

This Tissue Salt deals with the tension created by trying to react to, and cope with the expectations and demands of others and the world in general. The pressure to fulfill expectations and the fear of failure are very strongly felt and have their origins in childhood experiences. This is a fear of embarrassment, of exposure and the need to hide self-perceived inferiority. This produces some involuntary physical reactions, resulting in the depletion of this particular mineral. The depletion often manifests hot flushes on the neck, the face and blushing in various situations.

The embarrassment a person feels when experiencing exposure, or even worse, when being ridiculed or sneered at, results in the need for large quantities of Magnesium phosphoricum. This Tissue Salt is also responsible for the body's automatic functions, such as heartbeat, nerves, glands and digestion.

If a child gets told by its mother: 'Behave yourself, don't you dare embarrass me!' it means that the child's value system will become corrupted. Not only will the child have to cope with the situation, but also needs to handle the pressure of not embarrassing the mother. In truth, the child is being ignored because mother is only concerned about herself - 'What will others think of ME?' The child quickly learns to pay heed to whatever other people say and think. The importance of the child's feelings take a backseat or gets lost, resulting in disastrous self-esteem consequences for the child.

In all likelihood the child is repeatedly reminded of the undesirability of being conspicuous in any way. Perhaps the parent may say things like, 'If you wear jeans to the concert, you'll be conspicuous!' or 'Aren't you ashamed of yourself that you have a different opinion?' This leads to self-denial in favour of being ruled by other people's opinions. The child learns to suppress tears and may even feign laughter in unhappy or painful situations.

Achievement anxiety is also enormous here, and so is a suppression tendency. That is why Magnesium phosphoricum as a "hot 8" works very well for constipation (holding back). Anyone with this syndrome is intense, while hiding their deficiencies because of the fear that someone else could discover their shortcomings. Magnesium phosphoricum is helpful in this regard.

No 9 - Natrium muriaticum

Inflexible, rigid and stubborn - everything is the fault of others.

When a child behaves in a normal way, the showing of natural tendencies demonstrates a need to be recognised. However, a child who is constantly rebuked, adapts to please others. The child will forget personal needs and will 'play-act' to please the parents.

Once the child is fully integrated into these behaviour patterns the same conduct is expected from fellow beings and engenders constraint and false relationships.

Having been conditioned into adaptation and submission mode, the child will yield to and accommodate everyone else's expectations without questioning them. This is how a child harvests the craved approval and acceptance from other people by wanting to know, 'Did I do well? Was I good enough?'

Frequently it is the expectations other people (not theirs) that is being satisfied, and if this does not produce the desired appreciation, sulkiness and grumpiness will follow. This type of behaviour can be called 'posthaste prior syndrome' and results in becoming a victim of their own expectations. If the other person is not happy with the proffered performance (which may not have been requested), the subject will simply go into overdrive and try to perform even better, with the same results. These experiences will not prompt the person to open himself up and change - but rather distance himself from the others.

The term, "sniffiness" would be suitable here, as the Tissue Salt, Natrium muriaticum - is most effective for colds and flues.

This type of life model will gradually suffuse the person, and apart from an ever-growing resistance to change, will also lead to physical inflexibility. First there will be cracking sounds in the joints, which progressively escalate to rigidity and even immobility as in rheumatism and gout. Lack of joint lubrication (where everything becomes blocked and lacks 'oil') can also cause arthritis. Chronic arthritis is another sign of inadequate inner mobility, and stubbornness. The affected person is often not aware of his own rigid disposition and actions.

The ensuing stereotype behaviour patterns are also frequently showcased in the form of certain mimicry and gesturing under various circumstances, such as flicking back one's hair in an affected manner, to allow it to fall forward again, or to push one's chin forward, or to stand in a supercilious pose. These are all symbols of fixated and rigid action models, which are far removed from uncontrolled and free expression.

No 10 – Natrium phosphoricum

The 'acidic' one. Life is strenuous and serious, not playful.

This Tissue Salt is responsible for the balance of acidity and alkalinity in the body. When a child is not allowed to argue or defend itself, or perhaps told to shake the hand of someone not liked, or to behave like an adult with regard to table manners and the like, the child feels threatened. These compulsions and constraints are connected with the words: YOU HAVE TO. The child grows accustomed to doing all the things the adult requests, but will internalize a feeling of frustration. As an adult these feelings are connected to the words: You have to help me, otherwise you will not go on holiday. You have to do your work, otherwise they will retrench you. Everything is a strain with no fun or play. Of course this pressure and tension in the body causes lots of acidity, which needs a lot of Natrium phosphoricum.

A child who experiences many orders related to, 'You have to,' may over time develop a thick skin. Because of the over acidity, there will not be enough working agents available to deal with fat-metabolism. The fat will be stored, and the resultant obesity may be seen as protective armour. If the body is over acidic, the character is often 'acerbic' as well. This might show up as heartburn, gastritis, stomach ulcer, diarrhoea or skin rash. During puberty a young person experiences tension, causing a certain amount of acidity in the body.

Because the acidity leaves the body through the skin, the disturbed fat-metabolism shows up as pimples and blackheads which can easily result in acne. As acidity influences the entire metabolism, gout may occur.

People with high levels of acidity are very often exhausted and feel burnt out. Because most of the Tissue Salts are depleted, the cells are unable to build up a proper energy field. This is only possible if the cells are loaded with enough minerals. Due to hyperacidity, the body misses the necessary minerals for the neutralisation. This means that there are not enough working agents to react properly on injuries, resulting in wounds healing much slower. This phenomena can be changed by bathing in seawater, which is rich in alkaline minerals that can equalize the acidity, promoting quicker healing.

No 11 – Natrium sulfuricum

Angry - controlling.

This Tissue Salt is responsible for the functioning of the liver and gallbladder, which are connected to the emotions of anger and rage. If the liver is overloaded with waste and unable to break it down, the organism will retain the waste in a watery solution (water retention). This fluid strains the body as it sinks into the tissue, thereby bloating them, resulting in swollen hands and feet. In severe cases, the body finds a way to get rid of

this fluid waste by creating an 'open leg' (ulcers cruris). There might be other disturbances, such as sun allergies (blisters with greenish fluid), bedwetting (as a result of holding emotions in), Herpes and fever blisters (anger, rage) bluish-reddish nose (irritated green and blue), liver diseases (unlived hate) etc.

Most of these people are likely to have been brought up in repressive ways, causing reactive lifestyles. They do not learn to take an active and creative attitude in life and are prone to waiting until outer influences force a reaction from them. They feel as though their lives are dictated by others, and become resigned to that fact. These people refuse to take responsibility for their own lives and often feel like victims.

Parents often prevent their children from acting independently because they tend to regard this as insolence. It is far easier for parents to raise their child in restrictive ways, as it releases them from dealing with the child's protests and self-willed individualism.

These children learnt to say 'one' or 'you' instead of 'I'. The use of 'I' could be considered arrogant by some parents. The child will, or has to accept this attitude, thereby suppressing individuality, in favour of emotional survival. This in turn creates self-doubt to the extent that it becomes insecure about the acceptability of his wishes. Again the child, in order to survive, ignores its own feelings. A vicious cycle develops where its reliance on other people's opinions grows exponentially. The more dependent on others, the greater the degree of self-suppression. This progressive development causes powerful emotional blockages and uses large amounts of No 11 Natrium sulfuricum.

As a result of the inner anger, uncontrollable emotional eruptions are experienced, which may be directed against itself. These reactions may be suppressed in a bid for self-control.

Repression of feelings leads to a situation where a survival strategy has to be developed. The repression is experienced as a threat which generates tension. The person will see dangers everywhere, mistrust everybody, and be incapable of integrating with life in general. Tension demands considerable usage of energy (No 6 Kalium phosphoricum), causing breathing difficulty (No 7 Kalium sulfuricum), requires gritting one's teeth (No 6 Kalium phosphoricum), tensing one's muscles and feeling very cold (No 2 Calcium phosphoricum). Whilst deep-down in the psyche there is hate for all those who will not subject themselves to the same limitations (calling for the currently described mineral No 11 Natrium sulfuricum).

No 12 – Silicea

Likes harmony but not conflict - friendly with everyone, living for others.

With this Tissue Salt, it makes sense to examine the psychological childhood background. Parents often have high expectations of a child and will dish out punishment if those expectations are not meet. Some parents may say things like; 'I'd rather you'd never have been born. That would have saved us a lot of trouble.' This is the worst kind of psychological punishment a child can experience. But nevertheless, the child will try to satisfy every expectation and demand. Initially the child will manage to accept and handle these at the expense of inner conflict and self-denial. Gradually the child renounces its own life in order to comply with external demands and conditions.

This person tries to avoid any kind of argument or conflict. Outwardly they will be friendly and in harmony to prevent conflict. This in turn leads to a high consumption of this particular Tissue Salt. The need to satisfy and fulfil others expectations, somehow makes them happy.

Many of these people believe in the principle: 'Nothing works out without the right connections; no job, no financial support, no discounts, etc'. They will only connect with those who are useful to them, that is on the surface, as a true connection to their inner being would be the prerequisite for a genuine relationship with another. But this person is always there for everyone else.

This falls into the same category as trying to secure a mother's love by finishing one's food, although no longer hungry. And before Dad starts disliking me, I'll do my homework. Lest I lose Mom's love, I'll even study the profession that she wants me to, etc. This gives the impression that no one is actually interested in what this

person wants or desires. Later in life this leads to humiliating self-doubt, as he may consider himself of little worth. This could also be a mirror of a partner who also has a need for this lack of self worth. Another way that they may look at it is they need the partner to fulfil them, which is a total self-denial. They also feel that the best thing in life, is when the other is happy. These people don't know what they really want for themselves, or if there is anything they do want.

Silicea deficient people are constantly waiting for something (that is not there), and go through life with long antennas so as not to miss out. They are, after all, responsible for everything and everybody. Such an externally directed condition does not allow recognition of what is of no relevance for this person, and often leads to a feeling of having to be on call for all and sundry.

Case studies

Case Study 1

S.W a 54 year old woman with eye problems and impure skin asked for Facial Analysis. She was always tired and had disrupted sleep patterns. She had lived in the same room for 5 years. In that time her state of health deteriorated, but she didn't know why.

A Facial Analysis reading detected Hyperacidity and also strain as a result of electricity symptoms in her face. I felt it was necessary to check the bedroom. The measuring instrument for electric pollution indicated 25 Volts against the wall, just behind where her head rests! The highest tolerable measure of electricity in a bedroom is 0.5 Volt. The reason for the enormous electrical strain was that the switchboard for the electrical supply was situated in the next room, right above her head. She almost lost an eye because of this strain.

As she couldn't move out of her room, we had to find a solution. So, we pulled the bed 30 cm away from the wall and added a wooden headboard. Immediately her sleeping patterns improved.

After checking her nutrition, she accepted some changes. There were too many acid builders, such as meat, sweets, pasta and not enough balancing vegetables and salads.

To support this, she took a Tissue Salts mixture and is slowly recuperating. The first positive sign was that she is not so tired and has more energy and vitality.

Case Study 2

I.H was 58 years old and for a long time suffered from Thyroid Gland problems. After many years of taking the chemical remedies of Allopathic drugs, she stopped taking them. However, the problem was no better.

Facial Analysis revealed many mineral deficiencies and a hyperthyroidism and a bedroom check was positive and so we moved the bed to another position.

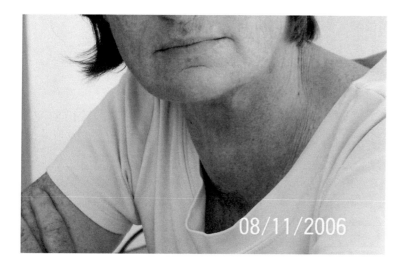

She took a large amount of Tissue Salts and recommended (related) Vitamins. It only took a month for the swollen thyroid gland to diminished in size. The reduction can be seen in the bottom picture.

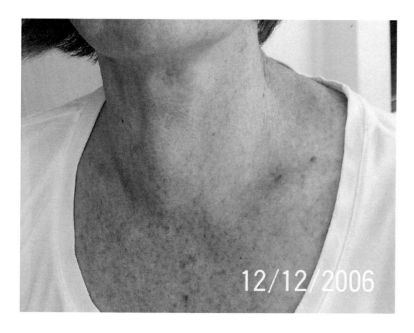

Case Study 3

I (the author) was deficient on all Tissue Salts, burnt out and with little vitality. For many years I lived in a house with lots of electro pollution in the form of field lines (water veins, earth grids and crossings, power lines).

After learning about Tissue Salts, I took 250 tablets a day for a year. Later I introduced some required vitamins and food supplements. Even if I did take vitamins and supplements, they would not have been absorbed due to the lack of minerals on a cell level.

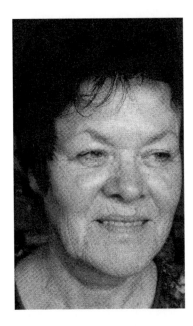

2004 – before Tissue Salts

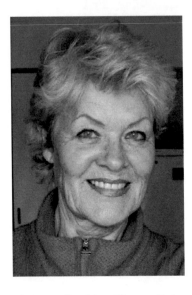

2009 - still taking Tissue Salts

Take Tissue Salts for health and get the face-lift for free!

Case Study 4

M.J. was constantly plagued with a red runny nose and so always carried paper tissues. She was easily embarrassed, which showed as violent red spots on her face and neck.

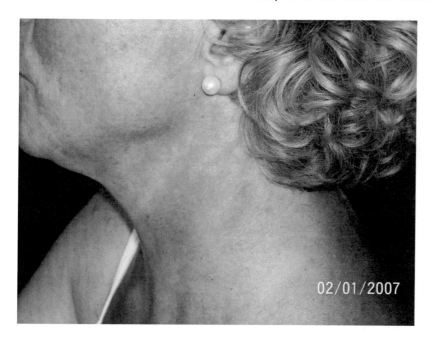

After taking a daily Tissue Salt mixture for 2 months, the nose is less runny (Natrium muriaticum) and the hectic spots (Magnesium phosphoricum) are diminishing.

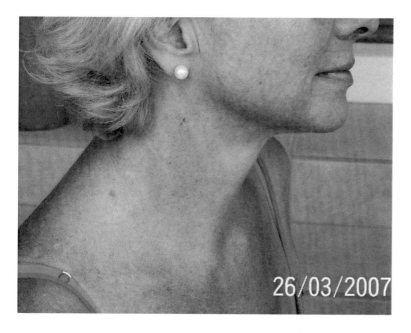

Case Study 5

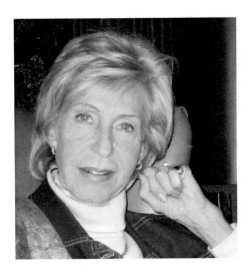

L. H, a very active and attractive business woman (64) had a chronic Iron deficiency. As a result she was always tired and suffered from cold hands and feet.

Twice a year she had to work at a fair for 3 days, but because of her energy breakdowns and could not spend an entire day at the show.

For many years she took iron pills, as advised by her doctor and did feel better as a result. But if she stopped taking them, the same symptoms returned and her blood count showed no improvement.

Facial Analysis showed the well-known Iron deficiency marks, and that her cells were depleted. She was also short of many other minerals. Her breakdowns of energy and cravings for sweets and chocolate are explicably due to the deficiency of No 10 Natrium phosphoricum. I gave her a balanced Tissue Salt combination including Ferrum phosphoricum, whilst she continued to take the Iron – but only half the amount.

After 6 months she did not require Iron pills. The Tissue Salts (on a cellular level) had stocked the cells, which meant that she was able to absorb the Iron. Her disciplined intake of Tissue Salts over a long period helped her to get rid of almost all her complaints. Today she is able to work the fairs for the three days without any breakdown of energy. Her craving for sweets decreased tremendously. She feels energetic and full of vitality and even has a new husband…

Case Study 6

Megan a hyperactive 7 year old craved sweets and chocolate.

The bedroom check showed bad radiation and Facial Analysis revealed that she was short of several Tissue Salts. She had a clear case of ADD (Attention Deficiency Disorder Hyperactivity).

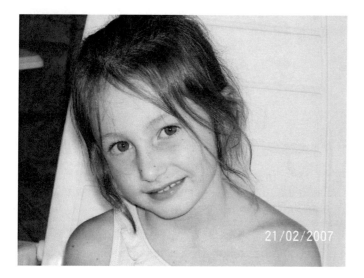

Only 4 weeks later; after taking the daily amount of Tissue Salts with related Vitamins, supported by an improved diet and a bedroom change, there were no more cravings for sweets, her sleep was more peaceful and her health in general is better. But more importantly she calmed down!

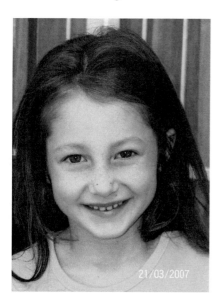

Case Study 7

Anonomous, a very active man (54) suffered pain as a result of an enlarged prostate gland. As a horse-riding teacher he needed to be pain free and was desperate to find a solution so as to avoid an operation.

Happily he took the recommended Tissue Salt mixture and after two weeks he called and was very excited about the fact that for the first time in years he was without pain.

Case Study 8

Calpe an old dog, recently had an accident where he had a broken thighbone. The vet inserted screws into the bone to hold it together. In studying the x-ray he noticed that the bone density (osteoporosis) was very low. As a result, the screws did not hold the bones. This meant that the poor animal had to be operated on a second time. The results could have been the same.

The desperate owner looked for a better solution and as she has taken Tissue salts herself, thought that she would try them. I gave her a tailor-made combination to improve the bone growth (osteoporosis).
Calpe loved the tablets and licked the paste from her owner's hand and also from his wound, on which Tissue Salts had been applied. Three weeks later the vet x-rayed the dog and saw that the screws were still in place. Dumbfounded he couldn't believe when he saw new bone tissue! The Tissue Salts had done their work and supported the healing process whilst building up new bone structure. After a few weeks the dog could walk. The owner was overjoyed.

Case Study 9

The 56 year old wife of a successful businessman informed me that over an 8 year period she had suffered from Diarrhoea. In addition, her blood pressure was high, she had a cough and in general was not well.

After the years of Diarrhoea her body was completely starved of minerals, which had implications on the cell level.

Facial Analysis confirmed her complaints and detected a few more. As she was taking blood pressure pills, I advised a slow start to her Tissue Salts intake, with the main Tissue Salt No 9 Natrium muriaticum which influences high blood pressure.

Three weeks of taking a Tissue Salts mixture cleared the Diarrhoea and so, after a time her whole organism started to regenerate, and she felt better and better.

Case Study 10

D.H, a 45-year-old Lady was never thirsty. When friends told here that she should drink more, she said. 'I can't,' which was true.

Clues in her face gave the answer, such as; red dry spots on the hairline, large pores and dry skin. The signs confirmed that she was short of No 9 Natrium muriaticum on a cellular level. The organism struggled with the intake of fluids because the cells didn't contain enough working agents (No 9) to assimilate the fluid.

During Facial Analysis I was able to demonstrate a working example of how Tissue Salts can help. I offered her 10 tablets of Natrium muriaticum and a glass of water. During the Analysis she had taken the Tissue Salts, but played with the water as there was still half a glass remaining. Drawing her attention to this, she took the glass and emptied it in seconds. She had not been able to do this for many years.

Case Study 11

A 41 year old lady (who was heavy with Rheumatoid Arthritis) wanted to join a group of runners who run 2 km every day. Her condition would not allow her to do this. During one of her meditations she asked for help and my name came up and so she called me for a Facial Analysis appointment.

The first thing we had to do was to detoxify her body using Tissue Salts, to reduce the acidity. The first few days she had taken the recommended mixture were awful for her. As with alternative remedies, it can happen that symptoms are aggravated before the healing takes place. But she carried on with the therapy and it is good that she did, as the symptoms slowly disappeared. The result - she was able to participate in the group and now jogs 2 k' every day!

Case Study 12

G.O. is an attractive 43 year old Yoga teacher, who suffered from a painful ear infection and Reflux. Facial Analysis confirmed many deficiencies. After only a few days of Tissue Salts, the ear infection was gone. She later announced that the Reflux has also disappeared - another success.

Case Study 13

V.E is a former elite athlete who exercised a lot. His face showed the classical signs of a sportsman: i.e. big pores!

Amongst other minerals, he was short in Natrium muriaticum (Water distributor). His face also showed a milky-purple discoloration which can be a sign of electro pollution. He was tired and did not have much energy, whilst his body produced a Phimosis (narrowing of the preputial orifice)

The shiny parts on his forehead and nose confirmed acidity (No 10 Nat phos). He told me that his working place was very close to high-tension wires. That means the body had to fight against this attack and used lots of No 5 Kali mur.

After taking the Tissue Salts combination for several weeks he felt much better. The extreme signs started to diminish, as well as the Phimosis.

Case Study 14

The man, now 55 years old, had had a By-pass. He suffered from a Melanoma and was a Diabetic 1. His face showed many different deficiencies and the body needed Tissue Salts urgently. As a Diabetic he had to dissolve and filter them. His body was completely acidic and I recommended that he change his diet and reduce his meat intake and eat more vegetables and salads.

Being keen to heal he gratefully took the advice and Tissue Salts. For a time he felt and looked better, but sadly after a short while gave up. His tendency for a lazy and sumptuous lifestyle was stronger…

Case Study 15

K.E is a very attractive lady and plays Tennis as often as possible. Suddenly she had her menses, not at the regular 28 days, but every week. Clearly there was something wrong. She did not want to go to the Gynaecologist because she was afraid he would give her drugs to suppress the symptoms. Of course being in her fifties she thought that she was at the beginning of menopause.

She asked for a Tissue Salt combination to stop the almost constant bleeding. After only 3 days, the symptoms completely disappeared. Six months has elapsed and she still takes the same mixture and has no more complaints.

Case Study 16

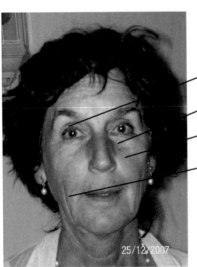

A.v.W complained about her brittle nails and tiredness. She is very attractive, but her hands showed dryness. When we met I discovered, that she also has other deficiencies on a cellular level.

No 7 Kali sulf

No 1 Calc fluor

No 5 Kali mur

No 12 Silicea

After taking the correct combination of Tissue Salts, 3 weeks later she called to tell me that her nails were beautiful and strong and in general felt much better, nor was she so tired. When I met her again, she did look much younger, fresher and more vital.

Case Study 17

A young woman, M.M. was constantly tired. I immediately saw that she was short of iron on a cellular level (even though her doctor had put her on iron tablets). I explained that if someone is mineral-deficient with iron on a cellular level, the intake of (macro) Iron as a food-supplement is useless, as the body can't absorb the iron. Here we would need an intra-cellular and extra-cellular balance. She took the advised Tissue Salt combination for iron deficiencies (micro) plus the iron, but only half of the quantity of the (macro) Iron. A few weeks later she looked much better and felt wonderful.

Finally the body was able to absorb the food-supplement and the tiredness disappeared.

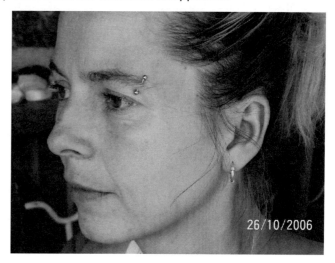

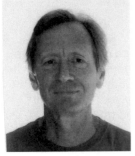

Case Study 18

B.G. suffered from migraines, was always tired and his eyesight was diminishing. Facial Analysis showed many deficiencies on a cell level, even though he ate quite healthy. He is a vegetarian but loved sweets.

The first thing was to help him with his sweet tooth, so as to reduce the acidity in his body. Tissue Salts are great for that (partly because of the lactose that tastes a bit sweet) and so for many people is an ideal replacement for sweets and partly because of the cell food. If the shortage of minerals is high, the body craves them. And interesting enough, the body knows exactly what food source to get them from. B.G. loved dark chocolate which contains magnesium. He was short of magnesium in the cells. When he ate the chocolate, he followed his body's need for magnesium. But this (macro) Magnesium from the chocolate used lots of (micro) magnesium in the cells to assimilate and digest the chocolate. By doing so, the deficiency in the cells increased and so the craving for the (macro) Magnesium increased accordingly.

This is the explanation for every craving we have, where different types of food require different Tissue Salts.

For a long time he was disciplined and took the Tissue Salts, which drastically reduced his sweet cravings. His body acid reduced and the tiredness decreased. In addition the migraines that he suffered from went. Then later, he started with a new mixture of Tissue Salts to treat his impaired eyesight. After a few weeks he was able to drive without glasses, something that he could not do for many years.

Case Study 19

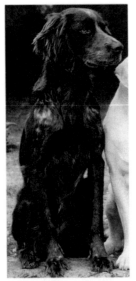

Lupa was a small 3-year-old German Münsterländer. She was very lively and jumped and played whenever she could. I found her at the age of 5 months – in fact, she found me… I don't know her past, but had the impression she had been a stray. Obviously there was not enough hydration as she had an extremely dry nose. This is not a good sign for a dog and usually means that the dog is ill. Fortunately she didn't have the health problems that are usually associated with a lack of hydration.

For a period of time I gave her (daily) 5 to 7 tablets of No 9 Natrium muriaticum – the water distributor. Occasionally I gave her the tablets to chew, sometimes I put them into her water bowl or sometimes dissolved them with a little water and mixed them with her food. It did not take long before she started drinking more water. After a few weeks, her nose was nice and moist! The water works in her body obviously was now balanced.

Case Study 20

A.M was visiting me one Sunday, simply to talk a bit. When she arrived, she asked, 'Do you have a pill for headaches?' I answered. 'I don't have any drugs in my household.'

Instead I offered her a "Hot 8" (10 tablets of No 8 Mag phos dissolved in half a cup of boiled water). She was sceptical and asked, 'Do you really think that will help?' Anyway she sipped the hot mixture and kept it in her mouth for a while. After 20 minutes she exclaimed that her headache was completely gone. I had a new Tissue Salts client.

Case Study 21

When I was playing a Tennis Club Championship game, my opponent (20 years younger and very fit) had just returned from a running competition. She was exhausted and I could have easily won. But that was not what I wanted, and after winning the first set, I offered her some Tissue Salts to recover. Gratefully she took some. Of course, I lost the following two sets!

As a result of her immediate recovery, she was convinced of the rejuvenating effect of Tissue Salts.

Tissue Salts are fast acting because they are absorbed by the laryngeal mucous membranes, from there the minerals go straight into the cells.

A TO Z GUIDE OF COMPLAINTS

Ailment / condition	Tissue Salts	Daily amount:
A		
Abdominal pain; bloating	Ferr phos No 4	10
	Mag phos No 8	HOT 8*
	Nat sulf No 11	10
	Cuprum arsenic No 19	5
	Kali aluminium No 20	5
	Nat bicarbonic No 23	3
Abdominal pain; colic	Mag phos No 8	HOT 8*
Ablactation	Nat sulf No 11	10
Abortion; imminent, threatened	Calc fluor No 1	5
(Additional to medical assistance)	Ferr phos No 4	5
	Kali phos No 6	10
	Nat mur No 9	10
	Silicea No 12	5
Abcess; in general	Calc sulf No 3	10
	Ferr phos No 4	5
	Kali mur No 5	5
	Nat phos No 10	10
	Silicea No 12	5
	Zincum mur No 21	5
Abscess; prevention	Nat phos No 10	10
Abscess; purulent, green discharge	Calc sulph No 3	10
	Nat phos No 10	5
	Nat sulf No 11	10
	Silicea No 12	5
Abscess; purulent, hardened	Calc fluor No 1	10
	Calc sulph No 3	10
	Nat phos No 10	5
	Silicea No 12	5
Acclimatization	Ferr phos No 4	5
	Kali mur No 5	5
	Kali phos No 6	5
	Nat mur No 9	5
	Nat phos No 10	5
	Nat sulf No 11	10
	Aurum mur No 25	3
Acid-alkaline balance; purgation	Calc sulf No 3	7

	Nat phos No 10	7
	Manganum sulf No 17	5
	Zincum mur No 21	5
	Nat bicarbonic No 23	3
Acidic tissue	Nat phos No 10	10
	Manganum sulf No 17	3
	Nat bicarbonic No 23	5
Acne	Ferr phos No 4	10
	Kali mur No 5	5
	Nat phos No 10	10
	Silicea No 12	5
	Zincum mur No 21	5
Acne; due to Contraceptive pill *(change product!)*	Calc phos No 2	10
	Calc sulf No 3	5
	Nat mur No 9	5
	Nat phos No 10	10
	Nat sulf No 11	5
Acne; due to puberty	Calc sulf No 3	5
	Ferr phos No 4	10
	Kali mur No 5	5
	Nat phos No 10	10
	Silicea No 12	5
	Zincum mur No 21	5
	Arsenum jodat No 24	5
ADD, ADHD - Attention Deficit Disorder *Attention Deficit (Hyperactivity) Disorder* *Change nutrition!*	Calc phos No 2	10
	Kali phos No 6	3
	Mag phos No 8	10
	Kali bromatum No 14	5
	Kali jodat No 15	3
	Zincum mur No 21	3
	Kali bichromic No 27	3
Aenemic children	Calc phos No 2	5
	Ferr phos No 4	7
	Kali phos No 6	5
	Kali sulf No 7	5
	Nat mur No 9	10
Agoraphobia *Air hunger (long term therapy)*	Kali phos No 6	10
	Kali sulf No 7	10
Alcohol; support with withdrawal	Mag phos No 8	10
	Nat mur No 9	5
	Nat sulf No 11	5
	Zincum mur No 21	5
	Selenium No 26	5
Alcohol intoxication	Nat mur No 9	10
	Nat phos No 10	5
	Nat sulf No 11	5
	Zincum mur No 21	5

Allergies; in general *(double the amount if necessary)*	Calc phos No 2	10
	Ferr phos No 4	5
	Kali mur No 5	3
	Kali sulf No 7	3
	Nat mur No 9	10
	Nat sulf No 11	5
	Zincum mur No 21	3
	Arsenum jodat No 24	3
Allergies; cats	Calc phos No 2	10
	Ferr phos No 4	5
	Kali sulf No 7	5
	Nat mur No 9	10
	Nat sulf No 11	7
	Arsenum jodat No 24	3
Allergies; detergent	Calc fluor No 1	5
	Ferr phos No 4	5
	Kali mur No 5	5
	Kali sulf No 7	5
	Nat mur No 9	10
	Nat sulf No 11	5
	Silicea No 12	5
Allergies; food refusal	Kali mur No 5	5
	Kali sulf No 7	3
	Nat mur No 9	5
	Nat sulf No 11	5
	Arsenum jodat No 24	3
Allegies; preservatives	Calc phos No 2	5
	Kali mur No 5	5
	Nat mur No 9	5
	Nat sulf No 11	10
	Arsenum jodat No 24	3
Alzheimer's disease	Calc fluor No 1	10
	Ferr phos No 4	5
	Kali phos No 6	10
	Kali sulf No 7	5
	Nat mur No 9	5
	Nat sulf No 11	10
	Silicea No 12	10
	Calc sulfur No 18	5
	Cuprum arsenic No 19	3
	Kali aluminium No 20	7
	Zincum mur No 21	5
	Selenium No 26	5
Amalgam fillings; elimination	Kali mur No 5	3
	Kali sulf No 7	3
	Nat mur No 9	7
	Nat sulf No 11	10
	Calc sulfur No 18	3
	Zincum mur No 21	3

Amoebiasis; amoebic infection	Ferr phos No 4	5
(Additional to medical assistance)	Kali mur No 5	5
	Mag phos No 8	5
	Nat mur No 9	5
	Nat phos No 10	10
	Nat sulf No 11	5
	Manganum sulf No 17	3
	Kali aluminium No 20	3
	Aurum mur No 25	3
	Selenium No 26	5
Anaemia	Calc phos No 2	10
	Ferr phos No 4	5
	Kali mur No 5	5
	Kali phos No 6	5
	Nat mur No 9	5
	Cuprum arsenic No 19	3
Anal eczema	Ferr phos No 4	5
(external use with similar Tissue Salts recomm.)	Kali mur No 5	5
	Kali sulf No 7	10
	Nat mur No 9	10
	Nat sulf No 11	15
	Kali arsenic No 13	5
Anal itching	Calc phos No 2	5
(external use with similar Tissue Salts recomm.)	Nat mur No 9	5
	Nat phos No 10	5
Anergy	Kali phos No 6	10
Angina; acute	Calc sulph No 3	10
	Ferr phos No 4	5
	Kali mur No 5	3
	Kali phos No 6	3
	Nat phos No 10	5
	Nat bicarbonic No 23	3
Angina; acute, purulent	Calc sulph No 3	10
	Ferr phos No 4	10
	Kali mur No 5	5
	Nat phos No 10	7
Angina; with bad breath	Calc sulph No 3	10
	Ferr phos No 4	10
	Kali mur No 5	5
	Kali phos No 6	7
	Nat phos No 10	7
Angina pectoris	Kali phos No 6	5
(Additional to medical assistance)	Kali sulf No 7	5
	Mag phos No 8 (often)	HOT 8*
	Silicea No 12	5
Anorexia	Calc fluor No 1	5

(Additional to medical assistance)	Calc phos No 2	10
(start with 1/3 and increase slowly dosage)	Calc sulf No 3	3
	Ferr phos No 4	5
	Kali mur No 5	5
	Kali phos No 6	5
	Kali sulf No 7	3
	Mag phos No 8	HOT 8*
	Nat mur No 9	5
	Nat phos No 10	5
	Nat sulf No 11	5
	Silicea No 12	3
Anti ageing; ageing process	Calc fluor No 1	5
	Kali phos No 6	5
	Nat mur No 9	5
	Silicea No 12	10
	Calc bicarbonic No 22	5
Ageing spots	Kali mur No 5	5
(also external application)	Kali sulf No 7	10
	Nat sulf No 11	10
Anti constipation; abuse	Calc fluor No 1	3
	Kali phos No 6	5
	Mag phos No 8	HOT 8*
	Nat mur No 9	5
	Nat sulf No 11	5
Antibiotics; stress in body due to abuse	Ferr phos No 4	10
	Kali mur No 5	5
	Kali phos No 6	5
	Nat mur No 9	5
	Nat phos No 10	5
	Nat sulf No 11	10
	Selenium No 26	5
Anti-oxidans (agent)	Ferr phos No 4	5
	Kali sulf No 7	5
	Nat sulf No 11	5
	Manganum sulf No 17	3
	Calc sulfur No 18	3
	Cuprum arsenic No 19	3
	Zincum mur No 21	3
	Selenium No 26	5
Anxiousness of children	Calc fluor No 1	5
	Calc phos No 2	3
	Kali mur No 5	3
	Kali phos No 6	5
	Mag phos No 8	3
	Nat phos No 10	3
	Silicea No 12	3
Anxiousness; due to inner restlessness	Mag phos No 8	5
	Kali bromatum No 14	3
	Kali jodat No 15	3

Appendicitis	Calc fluor No 1	5
(see GP!)	Ferr phos No 4	10
	Kali mur No 5	5
	Kali phos No 6	5
	Mag phos No 8	5
Aphta; white, stomatitis	Calc sulph No 3	5
	Ferr phos No 4	7
	Kali mur No 5	5
	Kali phos No 6	5
	Nat mur No 9	5
Appetite; loss of, chronic	Kali phos No 6	5
	Nat mur No 9	5
Appetite; loss of, with children	Calc phos No 2	3
	Ferr phos No 4	7
	Kali phos No 6	3
	Kali sulf No 7	3
	Nat mur No 9	3
	Nat phos No 10	3
	Calc carbonic No 22	3
Appetite; morbid	Nat phos No 10	10
Arteriosclerosis	Calc fluor No 1	3
(external use with similar Tissue Salts recomm.)	Kali mur No 5	3
	Mag phos No 8	5
	Nat phos No 10	5
	Nat sulf No 11	5
	Silicea No 12	3
	Manganum sulf No 17	3
	Cuprum arsenic No 19	3
	Selenium No 26	3
	Kali bichromic No 27	5
Arthritis; inflammed joints	Calc fluor No 1	3
(external use with similar Tissue Salts recomm.)	Ferr phos No 4	10
	Kali mur No 5	5
	Nat mur No 9	7
	Nat phos No 10	7
	Manganum sulf No 17	3
Arthrosis; deformed joints	Calc fluor No 1	3
(external use with similar Tissue Salts recomm.)	Calc phos No 2	5
	Nat mur No 9	5
	Nat phos No 10	10
	Silicea No 12	3
	Lithium mur No 16	3
	Selenium No 26	3
Articular pain; joints	Calc fluor No 1	3
	Calc phos No 2	5
	Calc sulf No 3	5
	Ferr phos No 4	5

	Mag phos No 8	5
	Nat mur No 9	5
	Nat phos No 10	5
	Lithium mur No 16	3
	Cuprum arsenic No 19	3
Articulation complaints	Calc fluor No 1	3
(external use with similar Tissue Salts recomm.)	Calc phos No 2	3
	Nat mur No 9	5
	Nat phos No 10	5
	Silicea No 12	3
	Calc carbonic No 22	3
Articulation; sound	Nat mur No 9	10
Articulation; swollen	Kali mur No 5	10
	Nat mur No 9	5
	Kali jodat No 15	3
Asthma; allergic	Ferr phos No 4	20
(Additional to medical assistance)	Kali mur No 5	5
	Kali phos No 6	5
	Kali sulf No 7	5
	Mag phos No 8	HOT 8*
	Nat mur No 9	20
	Nat sulf No 11	5
	Arsenum jodat No 24	5
Asthma; nervous	Calc phos No 2	5
(Additional to medical assistance)	Kali phos No 6	5
	Kali sulf No 7	5
	Mag phos No 8	10
	Nat mur No 9	5
	Kali bromatum No 14	5
Athlete's foot	Calc fluor No 1	3
	Kali phos No 6	7
	Nat mur No 9	3
	Nat phos No 10	3
	Nat sulf No 11	3
	Silicea No 12	7
Athlete's support	Calc fluor No 1	3
	Calc phos No 2	3
	Calc sulf No 3	3
	Ferr phos No 4	3
	Kali mur No 5	3
	Kali phos No 6	3
	Kali sulf No 7	3
	Mag phos No 8	10
	Nat mur No 9	10
	Nat phos No 10	5
	Nat sulf No 11	5
	Silicea No 12	5
	Manganum sulf No 17	3
	Zincum mur No 21	5

	Kali bichromic No 27	5

B

Baby bellyache; gripping pains in the bowel *(external use with similar Tissue Salts recomm.)*	Calc phos No 2	3
	Mag phos No 8	3
	Nat sulf No 11	3

Back pain; low back pain *(external use with similar Tissue Salts recomm.)*	Calc fluor No 1	3
	Calc phos No 2	5
	Ferr phos No 4	7
	Nat mur No 9	5
	Nat phos No 10	7
	Silicea No 12	3
	Calc carbonic No 22	3

Bad breath; even after cleaning teeth	Kali phos No 6	7

Bed wetting	Calc phos No 2	5
	Ferr phos No 4	5
	Kali phos No 6	5
	Nat mur No 9	5
	Nat sulf No 11	15

Belching; acidic	Nat phos No 10	7

Birth; weak contractions	Kali phos No 6	5
	Mag phos No 8	10

Blackheads, pimples *(external use with similar Tissue Salts recomm.)*	Ferr phos No 4	5
	Kali mur No 5	3
	Nat phos No 10	10
	Silicea No 12	3

Bladder; urinary incontinence	Nat mur No 9	5
	Nat sulf No 11	10
	Lithium mur No 16	3

Bladder; irritable, nervous	Calc fluor No 1	3
	Ferr phos No 4	5
	Nat mur No 9	10
	Nat phos No 10	7
	Lithium mur No 16	3

Bladder; inflammation	Ferr phos No 4	10
	Nat mur No 9	10
	Nat phos No 10	5
	Lithium mur No 16	3

Bladder; urinary urgency	Calc fluor No 1	3
	Kali mur No 5	5
	Nat mur No 9	7
	Nat sulf No 11	5
	Lithium mur No 16	3

Blisters; watery, itching	Nat sulf No 11	10

Blisters; at lips, mouth	Nat mur No 9	10
	Nat sulf No 11	10
Blistering	Ferr phos No 4	10
(external use with similar Tissue Salts recomm.)	Nat mur No 9	15
Bloating; with pain, colic	Mag phos No 8	HOT 8*
	Kali aluminium No 20	3
Bloating; with stinky winds	Nat sulf No 11	10
Bloating; with sense of fullness in abdomen	Kali sulf No 7	15
Blood with high uric acid level	Nat phos No 10	10
Blood pressure; high	Calc fluor No 1	5
(Additional to medical assistance)	Mag phos No 8	7
	Nat mur No 9	10
	Nat sulf No 11	7
	Kali jodat No 15	5
	Aurum mur No 25	5
Blood pressure; low	Kali phos No 6	5
	Nat mur No 9	5
	Nat phos No 10	5
Blood viscosity	Kali mur No 5	10
Bone; poor formation	Calc fluor No 1	3
	Calc phos No 2	5
	Kali phos No 6	3
	Mag phos No 8	3
	Nat mur No 9	5
	Silicea No 12	3
	Calc carbonic No 22	3
Bone; fracture, speed up callus formation	Calc fluor No 1	3
(external use with similar Tissue Salts recomm.	Calc phos No 2	7
after removing plaster bandage)	Ferr phos No 4	5
	Nat mur No 9	5
	Silicea No 12	5
	Calc carbonic No 22	3
Bone; pain in old fracture	Ferr phos No 4	10
	Nat mur No 9	5
	Nat phos No 10	7
	Silicea No 12	5
	Calc carbonic No 22	3
Breast feeding; poor milk	Calc phos No 2	5
	Kali mur No 5	5
	Nat mur No 9	5
Bronchitis	Calc phos No 2	5
(external use with similar Tissue Salts recomm.)	Calc sulf No 3	5

	Ferr phos No 4	10
	Kali mur No 5	15
	Kali sulf No 7	5
	Nat mur No 9	5
	Silicea No 12	3
Bruises	Calc fluor No 1	3
	Calc sulf No 3	5
	Silicea No 12	10
Bulimia	Calc phos No 2	10
(Additional to medical assistance)	Ferr phos No 4	10
	Kali phos No 6	5
	Mag phos No 8	HOT 8*
	Silicea No 12	3
Burn	Ferr phos No 4	5
(external use with similar Tissue Salts recomm.)	Nat mur No 9	15
Bursitis	Ferr phos No 4	10
(external use with similar Tissue Salts recomm.)	Kali mur No 5	5
	Nat mur No 9	5
	Nat sulf No 11	5
	Silicea No 12	3

C

Callosity	Calc fluor No 1	7
(external use with similar Tissue Salts recomm.)	Kali phos No 6	5
	Nat mur No 9	5
Caries prophylaxis	Calc fluor No 1	3
	Calc phos No 2	5
	Mag phos No 8	5
	Nat mur No 9	5
	Silicea No 12	3
Cardiotonic	Calc fluor No 1	3
	Calc phos No 2	5
	Kali phos No 6	5
	Mag phos No 8	7
	Nat mur No 9	5
	Silicea No 12	5
Cardiac pain	Ferr phos No 4	7
	Kali phos No 6	7
	Kali sulf No 7	5
	Mag phos No 8	HOT 8*
	Silicea No 12	3
	Lithium mur No 16	3
Cardiac palpitation strong	Lithium mur No 16	5
Cardiac palpitation strong; at night	Calc phos No 2	7
Cartilage; disorders (sound, cracking)	Nat mur No 9	10

(external use with similar Tissue Salts recomm.)

Cartilage; swelling (due to gout, rheumatism)	Nat mur No 9	10
(external use with similar Tissue Salts recomm.)	Nat phos No 10	10
	Silicea No 12	3
Cartilage; disorders due to overstress	Calc fluor No 1	3
	Kali phos No 6	7
	Nat mur No 9	10
	Silicea No 12	5
	Manganum sulf No 17	3
Cataract; grey	Kali mur No 5	5
	Nat mur No 9	10
	Nat phos No 10	5
	Silicea No 12	5
	Cuprum arsenic No 19	5
	Zincum mur No 21	5
	Selenium No 26	5
Catarrh; suffer from	Ferr phos No 4	5
	Kali mur No 5	3
	Kali sulf No 7	5
	Nat mur No 9	5
	Nat sulf No 11	3
Catharsis; purgation (spring cure)	Calc sulf No 3	7
	Kali mur No 5	5
	Kali phos No 6	5
	Kali sulf No 7	7
	Nat mur No 9	5
	Nat phos No 10	5
	Nat sulf No 11	15
	Silicea No 12	3
	Kali jodat No 15	3
	Calc sulfur No 18	3
	Cuprum.arsenic No 19	3
	Nat bicarbonic No 23	3
	Selenium No 26	3
Chemotherapy; tonic	Ferr phos No 4	20
	Kali phos No 6	20
	Mag phos No 8	20
	Nat mur No 9	20
Chest pain; sensation of touch	Ferr phos No 4	7
	Kali phos No 6	5
	Silicea No 12	3
Chest pain; breast feeding	Nat mur No 9	20
Chest pain; before menstruation	Calc phos No 2	5
	Ferr phos No 4	5
	Kali mur No 5	3
Chickenpox, varicella	Calc phos No 2	5

	Ferr phos No 4	10
	Kali mur No 5	10
	Kali sulf No 7	5
Childbed psychosis; puerperal psychosis	Calc fluor No 1	5
	Calc phos No 2	5
	Calc sulf No 3	5
	Ferr phos No 4	5
	Kali mur No 5	5
	Kali phos No 6	10
	Kali sulf No 7	5
	Mag phos No 8	5
	Nat mur No 9	5
	Nat phos No 10	5
	Nat sulf No 11	5
	Silicea No 12	5
	Kali jodat No 15	3
	Calc carbonic No 22	5
Children; teething	Calc fluor No 1	5
	Ferr phos No 4	5
	Kali phos No 6	3
	Nat mur No 9	5
Children; cramps all kind of	Mag phos No 8	HOT 8*
Children; cramps at night	Calc phos No 2	3
	Silicea No 12	3
Children; whiny mood	Kali phos No 6	7
	Nat mur No 9	3
Children's complaints; 1st stage – start	Ferr phos No 4	7
Children's complaints; 2nd stage – setting	Kali mur No 5	7
Children's complaints; 3rd stage – chronic	Kali sulf No 7	7
	Nat sulf No 11	3
Cholesterol level; high (reduce stress and change nutrition)	Mag phos No 8	HOT 8*
	Nat phos No 10	10
	Nat sulf No 11	5
	Kali bichromic No 27	5
Cholesterol level; low	Mag phos No 8	HOT 8*
	Kali bichromic No 27	3
Chronic rheumatoid arthritis; Polyarthritis	Calc sulf No 3	5
	Ferr phos No 4	5
	Nat mur No 9	10
	Nat phos No 10	10
	Nat sulf No 11	5
	Aurum mur No 25	5
Circulatory debility	Calc phos No 2	3
	Ferr phos No 4	5

	Kali mur No 5	5
	Mag phos No 8	7
	Nat mur No 9	5
Circulatory disturbance; legs & hands	Calc fluor No 1	5
	Calc phos No 2	15
	Ferr phos No 4	10
	Nat mur No 9	5
Claustrophobia; fear of being in closed spaces	Calc phos No 2	5
	Kali sulf No 7	15
Clavus; corn *(external use with similar Tissue Salts recomm.)*	Calc fluor No 1	15
	Nat mur No 9	5
	Silicea No 12	5
Climacterium; complaints	Calc phos No 2	5
	Mag phos No 8	5
	Nat mur No 9	5
	Kali arsenic No 13	3
	Kali bromatum No 14	3
	Kali jodat No 15	3
	Aurum mur No 25	5
Climacterium; hot flushes	Mag phos No 8	HOT 8*
	Nat mur No 9	7
	Kali arsenic No 13	3
	Kali bromatum No 14	3
	Lithium mur No 16	3
Climacterium; complaints genital organs	Calc fluor No 1	5
	Kali phos No 6	10
	Nat mur No 9	10
	Zincum mur No 21	5
	Aurum mur No 25	5
Coeliac disease; gluten intolerance *(Additional to medical assistance)*	Calc phos No 2	5
	Ferr phos No 4	10
	Kali mur No 5	5
	Nat sulf No 11	5
	Cuprum arsenic No 19	5
	Zincum mur No 21	5
	Selenium No 26	5
Cold; slight	Ferr phos No 4	15
	Kali mur No 5	10
	Kali phos No 6	10
	Nat mur No 9	5
	Nat phos No 10	3
	Nat sulf No 11	5
Cold, common; rhinitis	Ferr phos No 4	5
	Nat mur No 9	15
Cold sensitivity	Nat mur No 9	7

Coldness; sensation chronic	Calc phos No 2	10
Colicky pain	Mag phos No 8	HOT 8*
Colic; bloating, constipation (adults)	Cuprum arsenic No 19	5
	Kali aluminium No 20	5
Colic; bloating, constipation (babies, children)	Calc phos No 2	5
	Mag phos No 8	10
	Nat sulf No 11	5
Concentration; lack of, poor	Ferr phos No 4	10
	Manganum sulf No 17	3
Concussion of the brain (see GP!)	Ferr phos No 4	5
	Kali phos No 6	10
	Mag phos No 8	3
	Nat sulf No 11	3
Conjunctivitis; pink eye	Calc sulf No 3	5
	Ferr phos No 4	10
	Kali sulf No 7	5
	Nat phos No 10	10
	Silicea No 12	10
Connective tissue; weak	Calc fluor No 1	10
	Calc sulf No 3	10
	Kali phos No 6	10
	Nat mur No 9	10
	Silicea No 12	10
	Cuprum arsenic No 19	3
Constipation; chronic	Ferr phos No 4	5
	Mag phos No 8	HOT 8*
	Nat mur No 9	10
	Nat phos No 10	7
	Nat sulf No 11	7
Contraceptive; hormonal problems	Calc fluor No 1	5
	Calc phos No 2	10
	Kali mur No 5	5
	Nat phos No 10	5
	Silicea No 12	5
	Kali jodatum No 15	3
	Zincum mur No 21	3
Convalescence; after heavy illness	Calc phos No 2	7
	Ferr phos No 4	7
	Kali phos No 6	5
	Kali sulf No 7	5
	Nat mur No 9	10
	Nat sulf No 11	10
	Calc carbonic No 22	5
Convalescence; after pregnancy	Calc fluor No 1	3

(to refill the depots)	Calc phos No 2	5
	Calc sulf No 3	3
	Ferr phos No 4	5
	Kali mur No 5	5
	Kali phos No 6	5
	Kali sulf No 7	3
	Mag phos No 8	5
	Nat mur No 9	5
	Nat phos No 10	5
	Nat sulf No 11	5
	Silicea No 12	3
	Manganum sulf No 17	3
	Calc carbonic No 22	3
Cough; attack in the morning	Kali mur No 5	5
	Nat mur No 9	5
	Kali aluminium No 20	3
Cough; dry	Nat mur No 9	7
Cough; hacking *(external use with similar Tissue Salts recomm.)*	Calc phos No 2	7
Cough; mucous *(external use with similar Tissue Salts recomm.)*	Calc phos No 2	3
	Kali mur No 5	7
	Kali sulf No 7	5
	Mag phos No 8	3
	Nat mur No 9	5
Cough sligthly, hawk (permanently)	Kali jodat No 15	5
	Lithium mur No 16	5
Cough; spasm	Calc phos No 2	7
	Mag phos No 8	HOT 8*
Couperose (spider vessels) *(external use with similar Tissue Salts recomm.)*	Calc fluor No 1	5
	Kali mur No 5	10
	Silicea No 12	3
Cut (wound) *(first aid: external use as a paste or powder)*	Ferr phos No 4	15
Cut (wounds with slow healing)	Calc fluor No 1	3
	Calc sulf No 3	7
	Ferr phos No 4	7
	Kali phos No 6	5
	Kali sulf No 7	5
	Nat mur No 9	5
	Silicea No 12	3

D

Decubitus, bed sore *(external use with similar Tissue Salts recomm.)*	Calc fluor No 1	3
	Ferr phos No 4	10
	Kali phos No 6	10
	Nat mur No 9	10

	Silicea No 12	3
Dejection; depression slight ((autumn, winter)	Kali phos No 6	10
	Kali sulf No 7	5
	Silicea No 12	5
	Kali jodat No 15	3
	Calc carbonic No 22	3
Dementia; Alzheimer	Calc fluor No 1	5
	Ferr phos No 4	5
	Kali phos No 6	5
	Nat mur No 9	5
	Kali aluminium No 20	10
	Zincum mur No 21	5
Deposit due to acidity	Calc phos No 2	3
	Nat phos No 10	7
	Silicea No 12	3
	Lithium mur No 16	3
	Nat bicarbonic No 23	3
Desquamation; after heavy illness	Kali sulf No 7	10
Detergent; allergy	Ferr phos No 4	5
	Kali mur No 5	10
	Kali sulf No 7	5
	Nat mur No 9	5
	Nat sulf No 11	15
Detoxification purgation (spring cure)	Calc sulf No 3	7
	Kali mur No 5	5
	Kali phos No 6	5
	Kali sulf No 7	7
	Nat mur No 9	5
	Nat phos No 10	5
	Nat sulf No 11	15
	Silicea No 12	3
	Selenium No 26	3
Diabetes I mellitus (insulin dependent)	Kali sulf No 7	5
(Additional to medical assistance)	Mag phos No 8	5
	Nat sulf No 11	5
(See recommendation for Diabetes)	Manganum sulf No 17	3
	Cuprum arsenic No 19	3
	Zincum mur No 21	3
	Kali bichromic No 27	3
Diabetes II (nutrition dependent)	Kali sulf No 7	5
(Additional to medical assistance)	Nat sulf No 11	7
	Manganum sulf No 17	5
(See recommendation for Diabetes)	Zincum mur No 21	3
	Kali bichromic No 27	5
Diaper napkin rash, soreness	Ferr phos No 4	3
(external use with similar Tissue Salts recomm.)	Nat mur No 9	3
	Nat phos No 10	5

Diarrhoea; in general	Ferr phos No 4	5
	Nat mur No 9	10
	Cuprum arsenic No 19	3
	Zincum mur No 21	3
	Calc carbonic No 22	3
Diarrhoea; after greasy food	Calc fluor No 1	3
	Nat phos No 10	10
Diarrhoea; foul-smelling	Kali phos No 6	5
Digestion; weakness, chronic	Nat mur No 9	5
	Silicea No 12	3
Digestion; weakness due to nervousness	Mag phos No 8	HOT 8*
Digestion; weakness due to acid food	Nat phos No 10	7
	Zincum mur No 21	3
Discharge; brownish-yellow	Kali sulf No 7	10
Discharge; watery	Nat mur No 9	10
Disintoxication; in general	Kali mur No 5	5
	Nat mur No 9	10
Dislocation, sprain *(external use with similar Tissue Salts recomm.)*	Calc fluor No 1	5
	Calc phos No 2	10
	Ferr phos No 4	10
	Kali phos No 6	5
	Nat mur No 9	5
	Silicea No 12	5
Dizziness; due to bloodlessness in head	Ferr phos No 4	5
	Kali phos No 6	5
	Mag phos No 8	HOT 8*
Dizziness; bending down	Silicea No 12	5
Draught; sensitivity	Nat mur No 9	7
Driver's mixture; to avoid overtiredness *(also useful for long flights in airplane)*	Ferr phos No 4	5
	Kali phos No 6	5
	Kali sulf No 7	5
	Nat mur No 9	5
	Nat phos No 10	15
	Nat sulf No 11	5
Dupuytren's contracture; tendon shortening *(external use with similar Tissue Salts recomm.)*	Calc fluor No 1	15
	Ferr phos No 4	7
	Kali phos No 6	5
	Mag phos No 8	5
	Nat mur No 9	5
	Nat phos No 10	5
	Silicea No 12	5

Dysphagia; difficulty in swalllowing	Mag phos No 8	HOT 8*

E

Ear; high pressure	Nat sulf No 11	5
Ear; discharge brown-yellow	Kali sulf No 7	5
Ear; discharge green-yellow	Nat sulf No 11	5
Ear; discharge purulent	Calc sulf No 3	10
	Nat phos No 10	5
	Silicea No 12	3
Ear; discharge white	Kali mur No 5	5
Ear; pain	Ferr phos No 4	10
Ear; pain and high pressure	Ferr phos No 4	10
	Nat sulf No 11	5
Ear; tinnitus	Calc fluor No 1	3
	Ferr phos No 4	5
	Kali mur No 5	5
	Nat sulf No 11	10
	Silicea No 12	3
Ear; tinnitus: sibilant noise	Calc phos No 2	5
	Ferr phos No 4	3
	Mag phos No 8	3
	Nat phos No 10	5
	Silicea No 12	5
Ear; tinnitus: whistling noise	Calc fluor No 1	5
	Nat phos No 10	15
	Silicea No 12	5
Ear; tinnitus with the beginnings of dull	Calc fluor No 1	3
	Ferr phos No 4	5
	Kali mur No 5	10
	Nat phos No 10	5
	Nat sulf No 11	10
	Silicea No 12	3
Eczema; skin rash *(external use with similar Tissue Salts recomm.)*	Ferr phos No 4	3
	Kali phos No 6	3
	Kali sulf No 7	5
	Nat mur No 9	3
	Nat sulf No 11	10
	Selenium No 26	3
Eczema; female genital part	Ferr phos No 4	5
	Kali mur No 5	5
	Kali sulf No 7	10
	Nat mur No 9	10

	Nat phos No 10	5
	Nat sulf No 11	3
Elimination in general	Kali mur No 5	5
	Kali sulf No 7	7
	Nat mur No 9	10
	Nat sulf No 11	10
	Calc sulfur No 18	3
	Zincum mur No 21	3
	Selenium No 26	3
Elimination; waste, environmental pollution	Calc sulf No 3	5
	Kali mur No 5	5
	Kali phos No 6	5
	Nat mur No 9	10
	Nat phos No 10	5
	Nat sulf No 11	10
Elimination; toxins from medical drugs	Kali mur No 5	5
	Nat mur No 9	7
	Nat sulf No 11	10
Enema; to regenerate *(dissolve mixture in water)*	Ferr phos No 4	5
	Kali mur No 5	5
	Kali phos No 6	10
	Mag phos No 8	10
	Nat mur No 9	10
	Nat sulf No 11	5
Enema; purification after fasting *(dissolve mixture in water)*	Calc fluor No 1	3
	Ferr phos No 4	5
	Kali mur No 5	3
	Kali phos No 6	3
	Kali sulf No 7	3
	Mag phos No 8	5
	Nat mur No 9	5
	Nat sulf No 11	15
Enema; if constipated *(dissolve mixture in water)*	Ferr phos No 4	5
	Mag phos No 8	10
	Nat mur No 9	5
	Nat sulf No 11	5
Endometriosis; uterine *(Additional to medical assistance)*	Calc phos No 2	10
	Nat phos No 10	5
	Silicea No 12	5
	Aurum mur No 25	5
Energy; lack of	Kali phos No 6	10
	Manganum sulf No 17	5
Epilepsy; falling sickness *(Additional to medical assistance)*	Calc phos No 2	5
	Kali mur No 5	5
	Kali phos No 6	5
	Mag phos No 8	10
	Nat phos No 10	5

	Silicea No 12	5
	Manganum sulf No 17	3
	Cuprum arsenic No 19	3
	Zincum mur No 21	3
Eye; cataract, grey	Kali mur No 5	5
	Nat mur No 9	10
	Nat phos No 10	5
	Silicea No 12	5
	Cuprum arsenic No 19	5
	Zincum mur No 21	5
	Selenium No 26	5
Eye; conjunctivitis, pink eye	Calc sulf No 3	5
	Ferr phos No 4	10
	Kali sulf No 7	5
	Nat phos No 10	10
	Silicea No 12	10
Eye; dryness or watery	Nat mur No 9	10
	Zincum mur No 21	3
Eye; glaucoma	Kali mur No 5	5
	Kali phos No 6	5
	Mag phos No 8	HOT 8*
	Nat mur No 9	10
	Nat sulf No 11	15
	Silicea No 12	5
Eye; grey film	Nat mur No 9	5
Eye; hordeolum, stye	Calc sulf No 3	7
	Ferr phos No 4	20
	Kali mur No 5	10
	Nat phos No 10	7
	Silicea No 12	7
Eye; Lacrimal adenitis	Ferr phos No 4	10
	Kali mur No 5	3
	Kali sulf No 7	3
	Silicea No 12	3
	Zincum mur No 21	3
Eye; Light sensitivity	Silicea No 12	10
Eye; Macular degeneration	Ferr phos No 4	5
	Kali phos No 6	5
	Nat mur No 9	10
	Silicea No 12	10
	Manganum sulf No 17	5
	Zincum mur No 21	5
Eye; Oedema	Nat sulf No 11	10
Eye; overstrained	Calc fluor No 1	5
	Ferr phos No 4	5

	Kali phos No 6	10
	Nat mur No 9	5
	Silicea No 12	5
Eye; Pain due to strain	Calc fluor No 1	3
	Kali phos No 6	5
	Nat mur No 9	5
	Nat phos No 10	10
	Silicea No 12	3
	Cuprum arsenic No 19	3
Eye; Photopsia	Mag phos No 8	HOT 8*
	Nat phos No 10	5
	Nat sulf No 11	10
Eye; Red eye lids	Ferr phos No 4	10
	Kali mur No 5	5
	Nat mur No 9	5
	Manganum sulf No 17	3
Eye; Scintillate	Kali phos No 6	5
	Mag phos No 8	HOT 8*
Eye; Swollen	Nat sulf No 11	7
Eyesight; poor	Calc fluor No 1	3
(Additional to medical assistance)	Calc phos No 2	3
	Ferr phos No 4	3
	Nat mur No 9	5
	Silicea No 12	3
	Manganum sulf No 17	3
	Zincum mur No 21	5
Exam nerves	Mag phos No 8	HOT 8*
Exhaustion; corporal	Ferr phos No 4	10
	Kali phos No 6	5
	Nat mur No 9	5
	Calc carbonic No 22	5
Exhaustion; due to acidity	Nat phos No 10	7
	Manganum sulf No 17	3
	Zincum mur No 21	3
Exhaustion; heavy	Calc fluor No 1	3
(start with small amounts, increase slowly)	Calc phos No 2	5
	Calc sulf No 3	3
	Ferr phos No 4	5
	Kali mur No 5	3
	Kali phos No 6	10
	Kali sulf No 7	3
	Mag phos No 8	3
	Nat mur No 9	3
	Nat phos No 10	3
	Nat sulf No 11	3
	Silicea No 12	3

	Calc carbonic No 22	3
Exhaustion; in general	Manganum sulf No 17	5
Exhaustion; nervous	Kali phos No 6	15
	Nat mur No 9	10
Exhaustion; with weight loss	Calc phos No 2	7
	Calc sulfur No 18	5
Excitement	Mag phos No 8	HOT 8*
F		
Face; crimson	Mag phos No 8	HOT 8*
Face; greasy shiny	Nat phos No 10	7
Face; grey, livor	Kali phos No 6	10
	Cupr arsenic No 19	5
Face; pale	Calc phos No 2	7
	Kali aluminium No 20	5
Face; reddish-blue	Nat sulf No 11	10
Facial neuralgia	Ferr phos No 4	7
	Kali phos No 6	5
	Cuprum arsenic No 19	3
Fasting; enema for purification *(dissolve mixture in water)*	Calc fluor No 1	3
	Ferr phos No 4	5
	Kali mur No 5	3
	Kali phos No 6	3
	Kali sulf No 7	3
	Mag phos No 8	5
	Nat mur No 9	5
	Nat sulf No 11	10
Fear of heights; hypsophobia	Calc fluor No 1	5
	Calc phos No 2	5
	Kali phos No 6	10
	Mag phos No 8	10
	Silicea No 12	5
Fear of flying	Mag phos No 8	HOT 8*
Fear of flying; take off and landing	Kali phos No 6	5
	Mag phos No 8	10
	Nat mur No 9	5
	Silicea No 12	5
Fear of travelling	Mag phos No 8	HOT 8*
Febrile blister; Herpes simplex *(external use with similar Tissue Salts recomm.)*	Ferr phos No 4	3
	Nat sulf No 11	10

	Silicea No 12	5
	Selenium No 26	5
Feeling cold; inner cold	Calc phos No 2	5
	Nat bicarbonic No 23	3
Feet; humid & cold	Nat mur No 9	10
	Silicea No 12	5
Feet; perspiration	Nat phos No 10	5
	Silicea No 12	10
Feet; pronation	Calc fluor No 1	7
	Silicea No 12	5
Fever; high (over 38,8 °C)	Kali phos No 6	7
Fever; slight (until 38,7 °C)	Ferr phos No 4	7
Fever; during travelling, stress	Calc phos No 2	5
	Ferr phos No 4	10
Fever; sunburn, diarhoea	Ferr phos No 4	7
Finger; tendon shortening	Calc fluor No 1	5
	Kali phos No 6	10
	Nat mur No 9	5
	Silicea No 12	3
Fingertips; cracked, sore *(external use with similar Tissue Salts recomm.)*	Calc fluor No 1	5
	Ferr phos No 4	7
First aid	Ferr phos No 4	7
Fissures; rhagades *(external use with similar Tissue Salts recomm.)*	Calc fluor No 1	10
	Ferr phos No 4	5
Fish-skin; Ichthyosis *(external use with similar Tissue Salts recomm.)*	Calc fluor No 1	10
Flail joint; excessive mobility of a joint	Calc fluor No 1	7
Flatfoot *(external use with similar Tissue Salts recomm.)*	Calc fluor No 1	7
	Kali phos No 6	5
	Nat mur No 9	5
	Silicea No 12	3
Food adjustment; during holidays	Ferr phos No 4	5
	Kali mur No 5	5
	Kali phos No 6	5
	Nat mur No 9	5
	Nat phos No 10	5
	Nat sulf No 11	10
Formication; poor circulation	Calc phos No 2	10
	Kali phos No 6	5

Fracture tendency	Calc fluor No 1	3
(external use with similar Tissue Salts recomm.)	Kali phos No 6	5
	Nat mur No 9	5
	Silicea No 12	10
Frontal sinusitis	Calc sulf No 3	5
	Ferr phos No 4	10
	Kali sulf No 7	5
	Nat mur No 9	15
	Nat sulf No 11	10
Frost-bite	Ferr phos No 4	5
(external use with similar Tissue Salts recomm.)	Kali phos No 6	3
	Nat sulf No 11	10
Fungal infection; intestinal mycosis	Ferr phos No 4	5
Nutrition!	Kali phos No 6	5
	Kali sulf No 7	10
	Nat mur No 9	5
	Nat phos No 10	5
	Nat sulf No 11	10
Fungal infection; pedal mycosis	Ferr phos No 4	5
(external use with similar Tissue Salts recomm.)	Kali phos No 6	10
	Kali sulf No 7	5
	Nat mur No 9	5
	Nat phos No 10	3
	Nat sulf No 11	10
Fungal infection; ringworm of the nails	Ferr phos No 4	5
	Kali phos No 6	10
	Nat mur No 9	5
	Nat sulf No 11	3
Fungal infection; stomatitis	Calc sulf No 3	10
(external use with similar Tissue Salts recomm.)	Kali mur No 5	5
Fungal infection; vaginal	Ferr phos No 4	5
(Also sitting baths with 10 T. of each Tissue Salt	Kali phos No 6	10
long-term therapy)	Kali sulf No 7	15
	Nat mur No 9	5
	Nat phos No 10	5
	Nat sulf No 11	7
Furuncle; suppurate pimple	Calc sulf No 3	10
	Ferr phos No 4	5
	Kali mur No 5	5
	Nat phos No 10	10
	Silicea No 12	5
	Zincum mur No 21	5

G

Gall-bladder; disease	Ferr phos No 4	10
	Nat sulf No 11	5

Gall-bladder; Bile-stone	Ferr phos No 4	3
	Nat phos No 10	5
	Nat sulf No 11	10
Gall-bladder; Biliary, colic	Mag phos No 8	HOT 8*
Ganglion *(external use with similar Tissue Salts recomm.)*	Calc fluor No 1	5
	Silicea No 12	3
Gastric bleeding *(see GP!)*	Calc phos No 2	5
	Ferr phos No 4	10
	Kali phos No 6	5
	Kali arsenic No 13	3
Gastric reflux; Oesophagitis	Calc fluor No 1	5
	Mag phos No 8	5
	Nat mur No 9	10
	Nat phos No 10	10
Gastric ulcer *(see GP!)*	Calc sulf No 3	10
	Kali phos No 6	5
	Nat mur No 9	7
	Nat phos No 10	10
	Silicea No 12	5
Gastric discomfort; after heavy meal	Nat phos No 10	10
	Nat sulf No 11	10
Gastric; pressing pain	Nat mur No 9	10
Gastric pain; hyperacidity	Ferr phos No 4	5
	Nat mur No 9	5
	Nat phos No 10	10
	Manganum sulf No 17	3
	Zincum mur No 21	3
Gastric; upset of the stomach	Ferr phos No 4	5
	Kali sulf No 7	10
	Mag phos No 8	3
	Nat mur No 9	3
	Nat phos No 10	3
	Nat sulf No 11	3
	Nat bicarbonic No 23	3
Gastritis	Ferr phos No 4	7
	Kali mur No 5	5
	Mag phos No 8	3
	Nat mur No 9	10
	Nat phos No 10	10
	Kali arsenic No 13	3
Gingival bleeding *(rinsing mouth with dissolved Tissue Salts)*	Ferr phos No 4	5
	Kali phos No 6	10
Gingival growth	Ferr phos No 4	5

	Kali mur No 5	3
	Kali phos No 6	3
	Kali sulf No 7	5
Gingival recession	Kali phos No 6	10
Glands; growth	Kali mur No 5	10
Glandular swelling	Kali mur No 5	10
Globus pharyngis feeling	Mag phos No 8	HOT 8*
Gluten intolerance; coeliac disease *(Additional to medical assistance)*	Calc phos No 2	5
	Ferr phos No 4	10
	Kali mur No 5	5
	Nat sulf No 11	5
	Cuprum arsenic No 19	5
	Zincum mur No 21	5
	Selenium No 26	5
Gout ; in general *(change nutrition)*	Calc sulf No 3	5
	Ferr phos No 4	5
	Nat mur No 9	10
	Nat phos No 10	10
	Nat sulf No 11	5
	Silicea No 12	5
	Lithium mur No 16	3
	Zincum mur No 21	3
	Nat bicarbonic No 23	5
Gout; attack *(also external use with similar paste of salts)*	Calc Sulf No 3	10
	Ferr phos No 4	20
	Nat mur No 9	10
	Nat phos No 10	10
	Nat sulf No 11	10
	Silicea No 12	10
	Lithium mur No 16	5
Greasy food; aggravation	Kali mur No 5	3
	Nat phos No 10	10
Glaucoma	Kali mur No 5	5
	Kali phos No 6	5
	Mag phos No 8	HOT 8*
	Nat mur No 9	10
	Nat sulf No 11	15
	Silicea No 12	5
Great toe; hallux	Calc fluor No 1	5
	Ferr phos No 4	5
	Kali phos No 6	5
	Nat mur No 9	5
	Nat phos No 10	5
	Silicea No 12	5
	Kali jodat No 15	5

Grumpiness in the morning	Mag phos No 8	HOT 8*
	Nat mur No 9	5
Growth detardation	Calc fluor No 1	3
	Calc phos No 2	7
	Ferr phos No 4	3
	Kali phos No 6	5
	Nat mur No 9	10
	Silicea No 12	3
	Calc carbonic No 22	3
Growth; pain	Calc phos No 2	10
	Ferr phos No 4	5
	Kali phos No 6	5
	Nat mur No 9	5
	Calc carbonic No 22	3
Growth disturbance; corporal, kids	Calc fluor No 1	3
	Calc phos No 2	5
	Ferr phos No 4	5
	Kali mur No 5	3
	Kali phos No 6	3
	Kali sulf No 7	3
	Mag phos No 8	3
	Nat mur No 9	3
	Nat phos No 10	3
	Nat sulf No 11	3
	Silicea No 12	3
	Zincum mur No 21	5

H

Haematoma	Calc fluor No 1	5
	Ferr phos No 4	5
	Kali mur No 5	5
	Silicea No 12	10
Haemorrhoids	Calc fluor No 1	10
(external use with similar Tissue Salts recomm.)	Ferr phos No 4	5
	Kali mur No 5	5
	Nat phos No 10	5
	Silicea No 12	10
Hair; falling out of hair	Calc fluor No 1	3
	Kali phos No 6	3
	Nat mur No 9	5
	Nat phos No 10	5
	Silicea No 12	10
	Zincum mur No 21	5
Hair; alopecia, loss of hair, round	Kali phos No 6	10
(see GP!)	Silicea No 12	5
	Zincum mur No 21	10
Hair; brittle	Nat phos No 10	10
	Silicea No 12	7

Hair; dandruffs	Calc fluor No 1	5
	Nat mur No 9	10
	Nat phos No 10	5
Hallux; great toe	Calc fluor No 1	5
	Ferr phos No 4	5
	Kali phos No 6	5
	Nat mur No 9	5
	Nat phos No 10	5
	Silicea No 12	5
	Kali jodat No 15	5
Hand; cracked skin	Calc fluor No 1	7
(external use with similar Tissue Salts recomm.)	Ferr phos No 4	5
Hands & feet; swollen	Nat sulf No 11	5
	Manganum sulf No 17	3
Hands & feet; cold	Nat mur No 9	10
Hands; sweating	Nat mur No 9	5
	Nat phos No 10	10
	Silicea No 12	5
Hands; trembling	Calc phos No 2	10
	Silicea No 12	5
	Kali bromatum No 14	5
Hangover; after excessive alcohol	Nat sulf No 11	10
	Zincum mur No 21	3
	Selenium No 26	3
Hangover; prevention	Ferr phos No 4	7
(to take prior to the party)	Kali phos No 6	7
	Nat mur No 9	7
	Nat phos No 10	7
	Nat sulf No 11	7
Hay fever	Calc phos No 2	5
	Ferr phos No 4	5
	Kali mur No 5	5
	Kali phos No 6	5
	Nat mur No 9	10
	Nat sulf No 11	3
	Arsenum jodat No 24	3
Heel; cracked skin	Calc fluor No 1	10
Headache; in general	Calc Phos No 2	10
	Ferr phos No 4	10
	Kali phos No 6	5
	Kali sulf No 7	5
	Mag phos No 8	HOT 8*
	Nat mur No 9	5
	Nat sulf No 11	10

Headache; children after school	Calc phos No 2	10
Headache; dull after alcohol	Nat sulf No 11	10
Headache; due to strain	Calc phos No 2	10
	Mag phos No 8	HOT 8*
	Cuprum arsenic No 19	3
Headache; forehead	Nat phos No 10	5
	Silicea No 12	5
Headache; from neck	Calc phos No 2	10
Headache; migrainous	Mag phos No 8	HOT 8*
Headache; pulsating	Ferr phos No 4	10
Headache; tension	Calc phos No 2	10
Head; dandruffs	Calc fluor No 1	5
	Nat mur No 9	10
Head; sweating smelly	Silicea No 12	10
Hearing; impairment	Calc fluor No 1	5
(Additional to medical assistance)	Ferr phos No 4	5
	Kali mur No 5	5
	Nat sulf No 11	5
Hearing; impairment slight	Kali mur No 5	10
Hearing; disorder	Nat sulf No 11	10
Hearing; acute loss	Ferr phos No 4	15
Heart attack; after care	Calc fluor No 1	3
	Calc phos No 2	5
	Kali mur No 5	5
	Kali phos No 6	5
	Mag phos No 7	5
	Nat mur No 9	5
	Silicea No 12	5
	Calc carbonic No 22	5
Heart attack; prevention	Calc fluor No 1	3
	Calc phos No 2	5
	Ferr phos No 4	5
	Kali mur No 5	5
	Kali phos No 6	5
	Mag phos No 8	5
	Nat mur No 9	5
	Silicea No 12	5
Heart attack; after care	Calc fluor No 1	5
	Calc phos No 2	5

	Kali mur No 5	5
	Kali phos No 6	7
	Mag phos No 8	5
	Nat mur No 9	5
	Silicea No 12	5
	Calc carbonic No 22	5
Heartbeat; uneven	Mag phos No 8	HOT 8*
Heartburn	Nat phos No 10	10
Heart hurry	Calc phos No 2	10
	Mag phos No 8	HOT 8*
	Kali jodat No 15	5
Heat; exhaustion	Ferr phos No 4	7
	Nat mur No 9	10
Heavy metal poisoning	Kali mur No 5	5
	Nat mur No 9	10
	Calc sulfur No 18	3
	Kali aluminium No 20	5
	Zincum mur No 21	5
	Selenium No 26	5
Hernia; inguinal	Calc fluor No 1	3
(external use with similar Tissue Salts recomm.)	Kali phos No 6	5
	Nat mur No 9	5
	Silicea No 12	10
Hernia; umbilical	Calc fluor No 1	3
(external use with similar Tissue Salts recomm.)	Kali phos No 6	5
	Nat mur No 9	5
	Silicea No 12	10
Herpes simplex; blister (starting phase)	Ferr phos No 4	5
	Nat mur No 9	5
	Nat sulf No 11	10
	Lithium mur No 16	3
	Zincum mur No 21	5
	Selenium No 26	5
Herpes simplex; blister	Calc sulf No 3	5
	Ferr phos No 4	5
	Kali phos No 6	5
	Nat mur No 9	5
	Nat phos No 10	5
	Nat sulf No 11	10
	Zincum mur No 21	3
	Selenium No 26	3
Herpes genitalis	Kali phos No 6	5
(Additional to medical assistance)	Nat mur No 9	5
	Nat sulf No 11	5
	Silicea No 12	5
	Zincum mur No 21	3

	Selenium No 26	3
Herpes suppurating *(external use with similar Tissue Salts recomm.)*	Calc sulf No 3	7
	Ferr phos No 4	5
	Kali phos No 6	5
	Nat mur No 9	7
	Nat sulf No 11	10
	Silicea No 12	5
Herpes zoster: shingles *(Additional to medical assistance)*	Kali phos No 6	5
	Mag phos No 8	5
	Nat mur No 9	5
	Nat sulf No 11	7
	Selenium No 26	5
Hiccups	Mag phos No 8	HOT 8*
Hip joint; restriction of movement *(external use with similar Tissue Salts recomm.)*	Calc fluor No 1	3
	Calc phos No 2	5
	Mag phos No 8	5
	Nat phos No 10	10
	Silicea No 12	3
	Calc carbonic No 22	3
Hip joint; pain *(external use with similar Tissue Salts recomm.)*	Calc fluor No 1	3
	Calc phos No 2	5
	Ferr phos No 4	5
	Nat mur No 9	5
	Nat phos No 10	3
	Silicea No 12	3
Hoarseness	Calc phos No 2	5
	Ferr phos No 4	10
	Kali mur No 5	5
	Mag phos No 8	5
	Kali jodat No 15	3
Hormonal balancing	Calc fluor No 1	3
	Calc phos No 2	7
	Kali mur No 5	3
	Kali phos No 6	3
	Mag phos No 8	7
	Nat mur No 9	3
	Silicea No 12	3
	Kali arsenic No 13	3
	Kali jodat No 15	3
	Selenium No 26	5
Hot flush; climacterium	Mag phos No 8	HOT 8*
	Nat mur No 9	7
	Kali arsenic No 13	3
	Kali bromatum No 14	3
	Lithium mur No 16	3
Hunger; permanent	Kali phos No 6	10

Hyperactivity of children; ADD, ADHD *Change nutrition!*	Calc phos No 2	10
	Kali phos No 6	3
	Mag phos No 8	10
	Kali bromatum No 14	5
	Kali jodat No 15	3
	Zincum mur No 21	3
	Kali bichromic No 27	3
Hyperacidity; stomach	Nat mur No 9	5
	Nat phos No 10	10
Hyperventilation	Calc phos No 2	5
	Kali sulf No 7	10
	Mag phos No 8	HOT 8*
Hysterical attack	Ferr phos No 4	5
	Kali phos No 6	5
	Mag phos No 8	10
	Nat phos No 10	5
	Silicea No 12	5

I

Induction of labour	Mag phos No 8	HOT 8*
Infertility; female	Calc phos No 2	5
	Ferr phos No 4	5
	Kali mur No 5	5
	Kali phos No 6	5
	Mag phos No 8	10
	Natrium mur No 9	5
	Cuprum arsenic No 19	3
	Zincum mur No 21	10
	Selenium No 26	5
Infertility; male	Calc fluor No 1	5
	Calc phos No 2	5
	Ferr phos No 4	5
	Kali phos No 6	5
	Nat mur No 9	10
	Nat phos No 10	5
	Silicea No 12	5
	Cuprum arsenic No 19	5
	Zincum mur No 21	10
	Selenium No 26	5
Inflammation; acute	Ferr phos No 4	10
Inflammation; chronic *(Immune system!)*	Ferr phos No 4	10
	Nat phos No 10	5
	Zincum mur No 21	3
Intervertebral disk; complaints	Calc fluor No 1	5
	Calc phos No 2	10
	Ferr phos No 4	5

	Mag phos No 8	10
	Nat mur No 9	5
	Silicea No 12	5
Immune system; strengthening	Ferr phos No 4	5
	Kali phos No 6	10
	Kali sulf No 7	5
	Nat mur No 9	10
	Nat phos No 10	5
Influenza infect	Ferr phos No 4	10
	Kali mur No 5	3
	Kali phos No 6	3
	Kali sulf No 7	3
	Nat mur No 9	5
	Nat sulf No 11	10
Influenza virus *(see GP!)*	Calc sulf No 3	7
	Ferr phos No 4	7
	Kali mur No 5	5
	Kali phos No 6	10
	Kali sulf No 7	3
	Nat mur No 9	3
	Nat sulf No 11	5
Influenza; during summertime	Ferr phos No 4	10
	Kali mur No 5	10
	Kali phos No 6	10
	Nat mur No 9	5
	Nat phos No 10	5
	Nat sulf No 11	5
Injuries; first aid *(external use with similar Tissue Salts recomm.)*	Ferr phos No 4	10
Insect bite *(external use with similar Tissue Salts recomm.)*	Calc phos No 2	5
	Ferr phos No 4	5
	Nat mur No 9	10
Intestinal; flu	Ferr phos No 4	10
	Kali mur No 5	5
	Kali sulf No 7	5
	Nat mur No 9	5
	Nat sulf No 11	10
Intestinal: complaints with spasm	Cuprum arsenic No 19	5
Iron deficiency	Ferr phos No 4	10
	Kali phos No 6	5
	Manganum sulf No 17	3
	Cuprum arsenic No 19	3
Itching; spodogenous	Nat sulf No 11	10
Itching; salty, burning	Nat mur No 9	10

Itching; hyperacidity	Nat phos No 10	10
	Zincum mur No 21	3

J

Jaundice	Calc fluor No 1	5
(see GP!)	Kali phos No 6	5
	Kali sulf No 7	7
	Mag phos No 8	5
	Nat phos No 10	5
	Nat sulf No 11	10
	Silicea No 12	5
Jaw; block	Calc phos No 2	7
	Mag phos No 8	HOT 8*
Jaw; chew sound	Calc phos No 2	5
	Mag phos No 8	5
	Nat mur No 9	10
Jetlag; prevention, complaints	Calc fluor No 1	5
	Ferr phos No 4	10
	Kali phos No 6	15
	Mag phos No 8	5
	Nat mur No 9	5
	Silicea No 12	5
	Aurum mur No 25	5
Joint deformation (due to gout, rheumatism)	Nat mur No 9	10
(external use with similar Tissue Salts recomm.)	Nat phos No 10	10
	Silicea No 12	3
	Lithium mur No 16	3
	Manganum sulf No 17	3
Joint pain; feet and toes (due to gout)	Nat mur No 9	10
	Nat phos No 10	10
	Nat sulf No 11	10
	Silicea No 12	3
	Lithium mur No 16	3
	Manganum sulf No 17	3

K

Kidney; strengthening	Ferr phos No 4	5
	Kali phos No 6	5
	Nat mur No 9	5
	Nat phos No 10	5
Kidney; stone – prevention	Calc phos No 2	10
	Mag phos No 8	5
	Nat phos No 10	10
	Silicea No 12	5
Knee; pain	Calc fluor No 1	3
(external use with similar Tissue Salts recomm.)	Calc phos No 2	5
	Ferr phos No 4	10

	Nat mur No 9	7
	Nat phos No 10	7
	Silicea No 12	3
Knee; rheumatic pain	Nat mur No 9	10
	Nat phos No 10	5
	Silicea No 12	3
Knee; stiffness	Calc fluor No 1	5
	Nat mur No 9	5
	Silicea No 12	5

L

Labial angle; inflammation	Calc fluor No 1	5
(external use with similar Tissue Salts recomm.)	Ferr phos No 4	10
	Kali phos No 6	5
Lacrimal sack; swollen eyes, chronic	Kali sulf No 7	7
	Nat sulf No 11	10
Laryngitis	Ferr phos No 4	10
	Kali sulf No 7	5
	Nat mur No 9	5
	Nat phos No 10	5
	Silicea No 12	5
Legs; cramping calves	Calc phos No 2	10
	Mag phos No 8	5
	Nat phos No 10	5
Legs; heavy, swollen, water retention	Nat sulf No 11	10
Legs; ulcerated	Calc sulf No 3	5
(external use with similar Tissue Salts recomm.)	Kali mur No 5	5
	Nat mur No 9	5
	Nat phos No 10	10
	Nat sulf No 11	15
	Silicea No 12	5
Learning; difficulties	Ferr phos No 4	5
	Kali phos No 6	5
	Kali sulf No 7	5
	Nat mur No 9	7
Leukaemia	Calc phos No 2	5
(Additional to medical assistance)	Kali mur No 5	5
	Kali phos No 6	5
	Mag phos No 8	10
	Nat mur No 9	5
	Lithium mur No 16	5
Ligament; tearing of	Calc fluor No 1	5
	Ferr phos No 4	7
	Nat phos No 10	7
	Silicea No 12	5

Light sensitivity	Kali phos No 6	5
	Nat mur No 9	5
	Silicea No 12	10
Lips; blue	Calc fluor No 1	7
Lips; dry, cracked skin	Calc fluor No 1	10
(external use with similar Tissue Salts recomm.)	Kali sulf No 7	7
	Nat mur No 9	5
	Silicea No 12	5
Limbs; pins & needles	Calc phos No 2	10
	Silicea No 12	5
Limbs; pain due to acidosis	Ferr phos No 4	7
	Nat phos No 10	10
	Manganum sulf No 17	3
	Zincum mur No 21	3
Liver; complaints	Kali mur No 5	5
	Kali sulf No 7	5
	Nat phos No 10	5
	Nat sulf No 11	10
	Kali alumin No 20	3
	Zincum mur No 21	3
	Selenium No 26	3
Liver; spot	Kali sulf No 7	7
(external use with similar Tissue Salts recomm.)		
Lungs; emphysema	Calc fluor No 1	5
(see GP!)	Ferr phos No 4	5
	Kali phos No 6	5
	Nat mur No 9	5
Lungs; pulmonary embolism	Calc fluor No 1	3
(see GP, hospital)	Calc sulf No 3	10
	Ferr phos No 4	5
	Kali mur No 5	10
Lumbago; low back pain	Calc fluor No 1	3
(external use with similar Tissue Salts recomm.)	Calc phos No 2	10
	Ferr phos No 4	5
	Nat mur No 9	5
	Nat phos No 10	10
	Silicea No 12	5
	Calc carbonic No 22	3
Lymphatic gland; harden	Calc fluor No 1	10
(external use with similar Tissue Salts recomm.)	Calc sulf No 3	5
	Kali phos No 6	5
	Nat mur No 9	5
	Silicea No 12	5
Lymphatic gland; swelling	Calc phos No 2	5

(external use with similar Tissue Salts recomm.)	Calc sulf No 3	5
	Kali mur No 5	5
	Mag phos No 8	5
	Nat phos No 10	10
Lymphatic system; congestion, due to acidity	Calc sulf No 3	7
	Nat phos No 10	10
	Nat bicarbonic No 23	5

M

Macular degeneration	Ferr phos No 4	5
	Kali phos No 6	5
	Nat mur No 9	10
	Silicea No 12	5
	Mangan sulf No 17	5
	Zincum mur No 21	5
Malaria	Calc phos No 2	5
(Additional to medical assistance)	Ferr phos No 4	10
	Kali mur No 5	5
	Kali phos No 6	10
	Nat mur No 9	5
	Nat sulf No 11	5
Marginal blepharitis	Ferr phos No 4	5
	Kali mur No 5	5
	Nat mur No 9	10
	Nat phos No 10	5
	Silicea No 12	5
Mastitis	Calc sulf No 3	5
(external use with similar Tissue Salts recomm.)	Ferr phos No 4	5
	Kali mur No 5	5
	Nat phos No 10	5
Maxillaris sinusitis	Calc sulf No 3	5
	Ferr phos No 4	10
	Kali sulf No 7	5
	Nat mur No 9	10
	Nat sulf No 11	5
Measles	Ferr phos No 4	10
	Kali mur No 5	10
	Kali sulf No 7	10
	Mag phos No 8	HOT 8*
	Nat sulf No 11	10
Measles; after care, strengthening	Calc fluor No 1	5
	Calc phos No 2	10
	Kali phos No 6	5
	Nat mur No 9	5
Memory; weakness	Calc phos No 2	5
	Kali phos No 6	10
	Nat mur No 9	5

	Silicea No 12	5
	Zincum mur No 21	5
Menopause; hot flushes	Mag phos No 8	HOT 8*
	Nat mur No 9	7
	Kali arsenic No 13	3
	Kali bromat No 14	3
	Lithium mur No 16	3
Menopause; weak skin	Calc fluor No 1	5
	Kali mur No 5	5
	Kali phos No 6	5
	Kali sulf No 7	5
	Nat mur No 9	5
	Silicea No 12	10
	Cuprum arsenic No 19	5
Meniscus; injury	Calc fluor No 1	3
(external use with similar Tissue Salts recomm.)	Calc phos No 2	3
	Kali mur No 5	3
	Nat mur No 9	10
	Silicea No 12	5
Menstruation; complaints with headache	Ferr phos No 4	7
	Mag phos No 8	HOT 8*
	Nat mur No 9	5
	Nat sulf No 11	5
Menstruation; with colicky pain, spasm	Calc phos No 2	5
	Mag phos No 8	HOT 8*
	Nat sulf No 11	5
	Cuprum arsenic No 19	3
	Zincum mur No 21	3
Menstruation; complaints, irregularity	Kali arsenic No 13	5
	Kali bromatum No 14	5
	Aurum mur No 25	5
Menstruation; heavy periods	Calc fluor No 1	10
	Calc phos No 2	10
	Nat sulf No 11	5
Menstruation; intermenstrual bleeding	Calc fluor No 1	7
	Mag phos No 8	HOT 8*
	Silicea No 12	5
Mercurial poisoning; amalgam teeth fillings	Kali mur No 5	5
	Nat mur No 9	10
	Nat sulf No 11	5
	Calc sulfur No 18	5
	Cuprum arsenic No 19	3
	Zincum mur No 21	5
	Selenium No 26	5
Metabolism poor; activation	Ferr phos No 4	5
	Kali phos No 6	5

	Nat mur No 9	5
	Nat sulf No 11	5
	Zincum mur No 21	5
	Nat bicarbonic No 23	5
	Selenium No 26	5
Meteoropathy; sensitivity	Calc phos No 2	7
Migraine; at beginning	Calc phos No 2	10
(repeat every 15 to 30 min)	Mag phos No 8	HOT 8*
	Kali bromatum No 14	5
Milk; allergy, intolerance	Calc phos No 2	7
Milk crust	Calc phos No 2	5
	Nat mur No 9	3
	Nat phos No 10	3
Mood; depressive, whiny	Kali phos No 6	7
	Kali jodat No 15	3
	Zincum mur No 21	3
Morbus Basedow; thyroid disease	Calc phos No 2	5
(Additional to medical assistance)	Kali mur No 5	5
	Nat mur No 9	5
	Kali bromatum No 14	3
	Kali jodat No 15	7
	Lithium mur No 16	3
Morbus Bechterev; spinal fusion	Calc fluor No 1	10
(Additional to medical assistance)	Calc phos No 2	5
	Mag phos No 8	10
	Nat mur No 9	5
	Nat phos No 10	5
	Silicea No 12	5
	Aurum mur No 25	3
Morbus Hashimoto; thyroid disease	Ferr phos No 4	5
(Additional to medical assistance)	Kali mur No 5	5
	Nat mur No 9	5
	Kali brom No 14	5
	Kali jodat No 15	5
Mother's mark	Kali phos No 6	5
(external use with similar Tissue Salts recomm.)	Kali sulf No 7	7
	Nat mur No 9	5
	Nat sulf No 11	10
Mouth; dryness	Nat mur No 9	10
Mouth sores	Calc sulf No 3	5
	Ferr phos No 4	5
	Kali mur No 5	5
	Kali phos No 6	5
Mouth; stomatonecrosis	Ferr phos No 4	7

(ev. dissolve in water and drop in)	Kali phos No 6	15
	Nat mur No 9	7
Mucous membranes; dry	Kali sulf No 7	5
	Nat mur No 9	10
	Nat phos No 10	5
Mucus; clear	Nat mur No 9	10
Mucus; greenish	Nat sulf No 11	10
Mucus; yellow-brownish	Kali sulf No 7	10
Mucus; white	Kali mur No 5	10
Multiple sclerosis (MS)	Calc fluor No 1	5
(Additional to medical assistance)	Kali phos No 6	5
	Mag phos No 8	10
	Nat mur No 9	5
	Silicea No 12	5
	Zincum mur No 21	5
	Selenium No 26	5
Mumps; epidemic parotitis	Ferr phos No 4	5
	Kali mur No 5	5
	Nat phos No 10	5
Muscles; aching, stiffness	Calc sulf No 3	10
	Kali sulf No 7	15
	Nat phos No 10	10
	Nat sulf No 11	10
Muscle; myosclerosis	Calc fluor No 1	10
(external use with similar Tissue Salts recomm.)	Calc phos No 2	5
	Ferr phos No 4	3
	Nat mur No 9	3
	Silicea No 12	3
Muscles; prevention aching, stiffness	Ferr phos No 4	7
Muscle; twitching before sleeping	Silicea No 12	10
Muscular debility	Ferr phos No 4	5
(external use with similar Tissue Salts recomm.)	Kali phos No 6	10
	Kali sulf No 7	5
	Nat mur No 9	5
Muscle rupture	Calc fluor No 1	10
	Calc phos No 2	5
	Ferr phos No 4	5
	Kali phos No 6	5
	Nat mur No 9	5
	Silicea No 11	10
Muscular spasm	Calc phos No 2	10
	Mag phos No 8	5

	Cupr arsenic No 19	5
Myoma; muscular tumour	Calc fluor No 1	5
	Kali mur No 5	5
	Nat sulf No 11	10

N

Nails; brittle	Silicea No 12	10
Nails; flexible, splintering	Calc fluor No 1	10
Nails; ingrown and inflammed	Calc fluor No 1	5
(external use with similar Tissue Salts recomm.)	Ferr phos No 4	10
	Kali phos No 6	5
	Kali sulf No 7	5
	Silicea No 12	5
	Zincum mur No 21	5
Nails; ringworm	Ferr phos No 4	5
	Kali phos No 6	10
	Nat mur No 9	5
	Nat sulf No 11	3
Nails; runaround	Calc sulf No 3	7
(external use with similar Tissue Salts recomm.)	Ferr phos No 4	5
	Nat phos No 10	5
	Silicea No 12	3
Nails; white spots	Calc phos No 2	5
	Zincum mur No 21	5
Napkin rash, dermatitis	Ferr phos No 4	5
(external use with similar Tissue Salts recomm.)	Nat phos No 10	10
Nasal; adenoids, polyps	Calc phos No 2	7
	Ferr phos No 4	5
	Kali mur No 5	5
Nasal; bleeding	Calc phos No 2	7
	Kali mur No 5	5
	Nat mur No 9	5
Nasal sinus; inflammation	Ferr phos No 4	10
	Kali mur No 5	5
	Nat mur No 9	5
Nasal sinus; pain	Ferr phos No 4	5
	Kali sulf No 7	5
	Nat mur No 9	10
Nausea; due to effort	Kali phos No 6	10
Nausea; due to eating	Ferr phos No 4	5
	Kali sulf No 7	7
	Nat mur No 9	3

	Nat phos No 10	3
	Nat sulf No 11	3
Nausea; due to hunger	Nat phos No 10	10
Nausea; due to excitement	Kali sulf No 7	10
	Kali jodat No 15	5
Nausea; due to bad food	Kali mur No 5	5
	Kali sulf No 7	5
	Nat phos No 10	7
	Nat sulf No 11	5
Neck pain; occipital pain	Calc phos No 2	10
	Ferr phos No 4	10
	Kali phos No 6	7
	Nat mur No 9	5
Neck pain; with stiffness	Calc phos No 2	5
(external use with similar Tissue Salts recomm.)	Ferr phos No 4	10
	Mag phos No 8	10
	Nat mur No 9	5
	Nat phos No 10	10
Neck rigidity; high tension	Calc phos No 2	10
	Mag phos No 8	HOT 8*
	Kali bromatum No 14	3
Need for; craving		
Alcohol	Nat mur No 9	10
Smoked meat, Ketchup, Mustard	Calc phos No 2	7
Milk	Calc phos No 2	7
Nuts	Kali phos No 6	7
Salt	Nat mur No 9	10
Chocolate (dark)	Mag phos No 8	10
Sweets, Cakes, white bread	Nat phos No 10	10
Nervousness; extreme	Ferr phos No 4	5
	Kali phos No 6	7
	Mag phos No 8	HOT 8*
	Nat mur No 9	3
	Nat phos No 10	5
	Silicea No 12	10
	Kali bromatum No 14	3
	Kali jodat No 15	3
Neuralgia; nervous pain	Mag phos No 8	HOT 8*
	Nat phos No 10	5
	Silicea No 12	5
	Cuprum arsenic No 19	3
	Zincum mur No 21	5
Neurasthenic	Ferr phos No 4	5
	Kali phos No 6	7
	Mag phos No 8	5
	Nat mur No 9	5

	Silicea No 12	5
	Kali arsenic No 13	3
Neurodermatitis	Calc phos No 2	5
(external use with similar Tissue Salts recomm.)	Calc sulf No 3	5
	Kali mur No 5	5
	Kali sulf No 7	5
	Nat mur No 9	5
	Nat phos No 10	10
	Nat sulf No 11	10
	Arsenum jodat No 24	3
Night blindness	Calc fluor No 1	5
	Kali phos No 6	5
	Nat mur No 9	5
	Nat sulf No 11	10
	Silicea No 12	3
Night sweat	Kali phos No 6	5
	Nat mur No 9	10
	Nat phos No 10	5
	Silicea No 12	5
Nipple; mamilla, fissured	Calc fluor No 1	5
(external use with similar Tissue Salts recomm.)	Ferr phos No 4	7
Nipple; mamilla, sore	Ferr phos No 4	10
Noise; susceptible	Silicea No 12	5
Numbness sensation; tingling	Calc phos No 2	7

O

Obesity; as a habit	Kali mur No 5	3
	Nat phos No 10	10
	Nat sulf No 11	3
Oedema	Nat mur No 9	15+
Olfactory; diminish, loss	Nat mur No 9	10
	Zincum mur No 21	10
Operation; long-term preparation	Ferr phos No 4	5
	Kali mur No 5	5
	Kali phos No 6	5
	Magphos No 8	HOT 8*
	Nat mur No 9	5
	Silicea No 12	5
Operation; after-treatment, regeneration	Calc fluor No 1	5
	Calc phos No 2	10
	Ferr phos No 4	5
	Kali phos No 6	5
	Nat mur No 9	5
	Nat sulf No 11	5

	Calc carbonic No 22	5
Opression at night	Kali sulf No 7	10
Orange-peel skin; Cellulite *(external use with similar Tissue Salts recomm.)*	Calc fluor No 1	3
	Calc phos No 2	5
	Calc sulf No 3	10
	Kali mur No 5	5
	Nat phos No 10	10
	Silicea No 12	5
	Nat bicarbonic No 23	3
Organ sinking; heterotopia	Calc fluor No 1	7
	Silicea No 12	5
Osteoporosis *(external use with similar Tissue Salts recomm.)*	Calc fluor No 1	5
	Calc phos No 2	10
	Calc sulf No 3	5
	Nat mur No 9	5
	Nat phos No 10	10
	Nat sulf No 11	5
	Silicea No 12	5
	Nat bicarbonic No 23	5
Otitis media	Ferr phos No 4	7
	Nat phos No 10	5
	Nat sulf No 11	7
Otitis media; chronic	Calc sulf No 3	3
	Ferr phos No 4	7
	Nat phos No 10	5
	Silicea No 12	3
Ovarian pain	Ferr phos No 4	10
Ovaritis	Calc sulf No 3	10
	Ferr phos No 4	10
	Kali mur No 5	5
Overweight; tendency	Calc sulf No 3	5
	Kali mur No 5	10
	Nat phos No 10	7
	Nat sulf No 11	7
P		
Pain; in general	Ferr phos No 4	7
Pain; lightning	Mag phos No 8	HOT 8*
Pain; pulsating	Ferr phos No 4	7
Pain chronic; rheumatic	Calc phos No 2	5
	Ferr phos No 4	10
	Nat phos No 10	5
	Silicea No 12	5

	Cuprum arsenic No 19	5
Paleness	Calc sulf No 3	10
Paleness waxy	Calc phos No 2	10
Pancreas disturbances	Kali sulf No 7	10
(Additional to medical assistance)	Mag phos No 8	10
	Nat sulf No 11	5
Paralysis	Kali phos No 6	10
(Additional to medical assistance)	Nat mur No 9	10
(external use with similar Tissue Salts recomm.)		
Parkinsonism	Calc phos No 2	10
(Additional to medical assistance)	Kali phos No 6	10
	Mag phos No 8	5
	Nat mur No 9	5
	Nat phos No 10	5
	Silicea No 12	5
	Kali aluminium No 20	5
	Zincum mur No 21	10
Penis phimosis	Calc fluor No 1	3
(external use with similar Tissue Salts recomm.)	Kali phos No 6	5
	Nat mur No 9	5
	Silicea No 12	3
Permanent cold	Calc sulf No 3	7
	Kali mur No 5	5
	Nat mur No 9	10
Perspiration; acidic smelling	Nat phos No 10	10
Pes valgus; sprained ankles	Calc fluor No 1	7
	Calc phos No 2	5
	Nat mur No 9	5
	Silicea No 12	3
Pharynx burn	Nat mur No 9	7
Pigmentation mark; pigment disorder	Kali mur No 5	5
	Kali sulf No 7	10
	Nat sulf No 11	10
PMS; premenstrual syndrom	Calc phos No 2	5
	Ferr phos No 4	5
	Kali mur No 5	5
	Kali phos No 6	5
	Mag phos No 8	5
	Nat phos No 10	5
	Silicea No 12	5
	Kali arsenic No 13	5
	Zincum mur No 21	5
	Aurum mur No 25	5

Pneumonia; pulmonitis *(See GP!)*	Calc sulf No 3	5
	Ferr phos No 4	10
	Kali mur No 5	5
	Kali phos No 6	5
	Kali sulf No 7	3
	Nat mur No 9	5
	Silicea No 12	5
Polyarthritis; chronic rheumatoid arthritis	Calc sulf No 3	5
	Ferr phos No 4	5
	Nat mur No 9	10
	Nat phos No 10	10
	Nat sulf No 11	5
	Aurum mur No 25	5
Poisoning; toxication (chemical) *(see GP immediately)*	Kali mur No 5	10
Poisoning; toxication (biological) *(see GP immediately)*	Nat mur No 9	10
Polyp; multipolypoid	Calc phos No 2	10
	Nat phos No 10	5
	Silicea No 12	3
Power mixture; immune booster	Ferr phos No 4	5
	Kali phos No 6	5
	Mag phos No 8	5
	Nat mur No 9	5
Pregnancy; support substance of the child	Calc fluor No 1	3
	Calc phos No 2	10
	Calc sulf No 3	5
	Ferr phos No 4	5
	Kali mur No 5	5
	Kali phos No 6	5
	Kali sulf No 7	3
	Mag phos No 8	5
	Nat mur No 9	5
	Nat phos No 10	5
	Nat sulf No 11	5
	Silicea No 12	3
	Kali jodat No 15	3
	Calc carbonic No 22	3
Pregnancy; preparation for child birth	Calc fluor No 1	3
	Calc phos No 2	5
	Ferr phos No 4	5
	Kali mur No 5	5
	Mag phos No 8	10
	Nat mur No 9	5
	Nat sulf No 11	5
	Silicea No 12	3
	Kali arsenic No 13	3
	Cuprum arsenic No 19	3
	Calc carbonic No 22	3

Pregnancy; Convalescence after pregnancy *(to refill the depots)*	Calc fluor No 1	3
	Calc phos No 2	5
	Calc sulf No 3	3
	Ferr phos No 4	5
	Kali mur No 5	5
	Kali phos No 6	5
	Kali sulf No 7	3
	Mag phos No 8	5
	Nat mur No 9	5
	Nat phos No 10	5
	Nat sulf No 11	5
	Silicea No 12	3
	Manganum sulf No 17	3
	Calc carbonic No 22	3
Pregnancy; vomiting	Ferr phos No 4	3
	Kali phos No 6	7
	Nat mur No 9	5
	Nat phos No 10	3
Pregnancy; Stretch marks *(external use with similar Tissue Salts recomm.)*	Calc fluor No 1	10
	Silicea No 12	10
Premature infant; support	Ferr phos No 4	3
	Kali phos No 6	3
	Nat mur No 9	3
	Cuprum arsenic No 19	3
Prostate; enlargement	Calc fluor No 1	3
	Mag phos No 8	10
	Nat mur No 9	5
	Nat sulf No 11	3
Prostate; inflammed	Ferr phos No 4	10
	Kali mur No 5	5
	Nat phos No 10	10
Prostatic adenoma	Calc fluor No 1	3
	Kali mur No 5	10
	Kali phos No 6	5
	Nat sulf No 11	5
	Kali jodat No 15	3
Prostatic cancer *(Additional to medical assistance)*	Calc fluor No 1	3
	Calc phos No 2	5
	Kali phos No 6	5
	Nat mur No 9	5
	Nat phos No 10	10
	Silicea No 12	5
Pruritus; in general	Mag phos No 8	HOT 8*
Pruritus; anal *(external use with similar Tissue Salts recomm.)*	Kali sulf No 7	7
	Nat mur No 9	5
	Nat phos No 10	10

	Nat sulf No 11	10
Pseudocroup *(see GP!)* *First aid: open windows, hang up damp towels*	Calc phos No 2	5
	Ferr phos No 4	5
	Mag phos No 8	HOT 8*
	Nat mur No 9	10
Psoriasis *(external use with similar Tissue Salts recomm.)*	Calc sulf No 3	5
	Kali sulf No 7	10
	Mag phos No 8	5
	Nat mur No 9	5
	Nat sulf No 11	5
	Lithium mur No 16	3
	Selenium No 26	5
Pulmonary embolism *(see GP, hospital)*	Calc fluor No 1	5
	Calc sulf No 3	10
	Ferr phos No 4	5
	Kali mur No 5	10
Pulse acceleration	Calc phos No 2	7
Purulent cavity; closed	Nat phos No 10	10
	Silicea No 12	7
Pus formation; chronic	Calc sulf No 3	10
Q		
Quinsy	Ferr phos No 4	7
R		
Rachitis	Calc phos No 2	10
	Nat mur No 9	5
	Nat phos No 10	5
	Silicea No 12	5
	Calc carbonic No 22	5
Rash; purulent	Calc sulph No 3	10
	Nat phos No 10	5
	Silicea No 12	3
Reconstituent; to improve fitness	Calc fluor No 1	5
	Calc phos No 2	5
	Ferr phos No 4	10
	Kali mur No 5	5
	Kali phos No 6	10
	Mag phos No 8	HOT 8*
	Nat mur No 9	5
	Nat phos No 10	5
	Silicea No 12	5
	Kali jodat No 15	3
	Calc carbonic No 22	3
Regeneration; after heavy illness	Calc phos No 2	7

	Ferr phos No 4	7
	Kali phos No 6	5
	Kali sulf No 7	5
	Nat mur No 9	10
	Nat sulf No 11	10
	Calc carbonic No 22	5
Regeneration; after operation	Calc phos No 2	5
	Ferr phos No 4	10
	Kali mur No 5	10
	Kali phos No 6	10
	Nat mur No 9	10
	Nat sulf No 11	10
	Calc carbonic No 22	5
Regeneration; after shock, shock therapy	Calc phos No 2	5
	Calc sulf No 3	10
	Ferr phos No 4	5
	Kali phos No 6	10
	Nat mur No 9	5
	Calc carbonic No 22	5
Resistance; synthesis	Calc fluor No 1	3
	Calc phos No 2	5
	Ferr phos No 4	3
	Kali mur No 5	3
	Kali phos No 6	3
	Kali sulf No 7	3
	Nat mur No 9	3
	Nat sulf No 11	3
	Silicea No 12	3
	Kali jodat No 15	3
	Calc carbonic No 22	3
Restless legs	Calc phos No 2	5
	Mag phos No 8	HOT 8*
	Nat phos No 10	10
	Silicea No 12	7
	Kali bromat No 14	7
	Cuprum arsenic No 19	7
	Zincum mur No 21	5
Restlessness	Kali bromatum No 14	3
	Zincum mur No 21	5
Rheumatism; in general	Calc sulf No 3	5
	Nat mur No 9	5
	Nat phos No 10	10
	Lithium mur No 16	3
	Manganum sulf No 17	3
	Cuprum arsenic No 19	3
	Zincum mur No 21	5
	Aurum mur No 25	3
Rheumatism; articulation, muscle *(external use with similar Tissue Salts recomm.)*	Calc sulf No 3	5
	Ferr phos No 4	5

	Kali mur No 5	5
	Nat mur No 9	10
	Nat phos No 10	10
	Silicea No 12	5
	Lithium mur No 16	3
Ribs, costal bone; bruise	Ferr phos No 4	10
(external use with similar Tissue Salts recomm.)	Kali phos No 6	10
	Nat mur No 9	10
Rosacea	Calc sulf No 3	5
	Ferr phos No 4	10
	Kali mur No 5	10
	Nat phos No 10	5
	Nat sulf No 11	10
	Nat bicarbonic No 23	5
Rubella; German measles	Calc phos No 2	10
(external use with similar Tissue Salts recomm.)	Calc sulf No 3	7
	Ferr phos No 4	7
	Nat phos No 10	5
	Nat sulf No 11	5

S

Saliva; stringy	Kali mur No 5	10
Saliva; poor, dry mouth	Nat mur No 9	7
Saliva; excessive	Nat mur No 9	7
Scaling; furfuraceous, yellow-brownish	Kali sulf No 7	10
Scarlet fever; with swollen glands	Calc phos No 2	5
(see GP!)	Calc sulf No 3	5
	Kali mur No 5	10
	Kali phos No 6	5
	Mag phos No 8	5
	Nat mur No 9	5
	Nat phos No 10	5
Scarring; hardened	Calc fluor No 1	10
(external use with similar Tissue Salts recomm.)	Kali phos No 6	5
	Nat mur No 9	5
	Silicea No 12	3
Sciatic pain	Calc fluor No 1	5
(external use with similar Tissue Salts recomm.)	Calc phos No 2	5
	Ferr phos No 4	5
	Nat mur No 9	5
	Nat phos No 10	10
	Silicea No 12	10
	Cuprum arsenic No 19	5
Sclerosis	Calc fluor No 1	5
	Kali phos No 6	5
	Nat mur No 9	5

	Nat phos No 10	10
	Silicea No 12	5
	Lithium mur No 16	5
	Mangan sulf No 17	3
	Cuprum arsenic No 19	3
	Calc carbonic No 22	3
Seasickness; prevention	Ferr phos No 4	5
	Kali phos No 6	10
	Mag phos No 8	10
	Nat phos No 10	5
Secretion; caustic, burning	Nat mur No 9	10
Secretion; itching	Nat sulf No 11	10
Secretion; brownish-yellow	Kali sulf No 7	10
Secretion; purulent, thick, yellow	Calc sulph No 3	10
	Nat phos No 10	10
	Silicea No 12	10
Secretion; purulent, watery	Calc sulph No 3	10
	Nat sulf No 11	5
	Silicea No 12	5
Secretion; watery clear	Nat mur No 9	10
Secretion; greenish	Nat sulf No 11	10
Secretion; salty, burning	Nat mur No 9	10
Secretion; acidic, sharp	Nat phos No 10	10
Secretion; watery, slimy	Nat mur No 9	10
Secretion; whity	Kal mur No 5	10
Shingles: herpes zoster	Kali phos No 6	5
	Mag phos No 8	5
	Nat mur No 9	5
	Nat sulf No 11	7
	Selenium No 26	5
Shiver; feel cold with fever	Ferr phos No 4	5
	Nat mur No 9	5
Shivers	Calc phos No 2	5
	Ferr phos No 4	10
	Kali phos No 6	5
	Nat sulf No 11	5
Shock; in general	Calc phos No 2	10
	Calc sulf No 3	10
	Ferr phos No 4	5
	Mag phos No 8	5

Sinusitis maxillaris	Calc sulf No 3	5
	Ferr phos No 4	10
	Kali sulf No 7	5
	Nat mur No 9	10
	Nat sulf No 11	5
Skin; impure, blackheads	Ferr phos No 4	5
	Kali mur No 5	3
	Nat phos No 10	7
	Silicea No 12	3
Skin; callus	Calc fluor No 1	7
Skin; cracked, fissured	Calc fluor No 1	7
Skin; dry, low moisture	Nat mur No 9	7
	Kali jodat No 15	5
Skin; dry low grease, strained	Nat phos No 10	7
Skin; dry, rough	Calc fluor No 1	3
	Nat mur No 9	5
	Nat phos No 10	5
	Nat bicarbonic No 23	3
Skin; rash itching	Kali sulf No 7	5
	Mag phos No 8	5
	Nat sulf No 11	10
	Kali arsenic No 13	3
Skin; yellow-brownish spots	Kali sulf No 7	5
	Nat sulf No 11	7
Skin; support and nutrition	Calc fluor No 1	3
	Ferr phos No 4	5
	Kali mur No 5	5
	Kali sulf No 7	5
	Nat mur No 9	5
	Nat phos No 10	5
	Nat sulf No 11	5
	Silicea No 12	5
	Cuprum arsenic No 19	5
	Zincum mur No 21	5
Sleep; disorders of initiating sleep, tension *(take all tablets together HOT)*	Calc phos No 2	3
	Mag phos No 8	5
	Kali bromatum No 14	3
	Zincum mur No 21	3
Sleep; disorders, irregular heart beat	Calc phos No 2	7
Sleep disorders	Calc phos No 2	7
	Mag phos No 8	HOT 8*
Sleeplessness; restless	Calc phos No 2	5

(take all tablets as a HOT drink: see HOT 8)	Kali phos No 6	5
	Mag phos No 8	5
	Kali bromatum No 14	5
	Zincum mur No 21	5
Slimming; reduction of hunger	Mag phos No 8	HOT 8*
	Nat phos No 10	10
	Nat sulf No 11	7
	Kali bichromic No 27	5
Smoker's cough	Ferr phos No 4	5
	Kali mur No 5	5
	Kali sulf No 7	10
	Nat sulf No 11	5
Smoking; support withdrawal	Mag phos No 8	HOT 8*
	Nat mur No 9	5
	Nat sulf No 11	10
Solar eczema	Calc sulf No 3	7
	Kali sulf No 7	5
	Nat sulf No 11	10
	Kali arsenic No 13	5
Soor; candidiasis	Calc sulf No 3	7
(external use with similar Tissue Salts recomm.)	Kali mur No 5	5
Spasm; colicky pain	Mag phos No 8	HOT 8*
Spasm; muscles	Calc phos No 2	7
	Nat phos No 10	5
Sports medicine	Kali sulf No 7	3
	Mag phos No 8	5
	Nat phos No 10	5
	Nat sulf No 11	3
	Manganum sulf No 17	3
	Zinc chlor No 21	3
	Kali bichromic No 27	3
Springtime rhinitis	Ferr phos No 4	5
	Kali sulf No 7	5
	Nat mur No 9	5
	Nat sulf No 11	10
Springtime tiredness	Calc sulf No 3	5
	Ferr phos No 4	5
	Kali phos No 6	10
	Kali sulf No 7	5
	Nat phos No 10	5
	Nat sulf No 11	7
	Silicea No 12	5
Spider veins; spider bursts	Calc fluor No 1	5
(external use with similar Tissue Salts recomm.)	Kali mur No 5	10
	Nat phos No 10	5

	Silicea No 12	5
Squint; strabismus	Calc phos No 2	10
	Kali phos No 6	5
	Mag phos No 8	5
	Nat mur No 9	5
	Nat phos No 10	5
Stage fright	Mag phos No 8	HOT 8*
Stitch	Mag phos No 8	HOT 8*
Stones; kidneys, formation due to acidity	Calc phos No 2	5
	Mag phos No 8	5
	Nat phos No 10	10
	Silicea No 12	5
Stool biliary; chronic	Nat sulf No 11	7
Stool; greasy	Calc fluor No 1	3
	Nat phos No 10	10
Strain; muscle, tendon *(external use with similar Tissue Salts recomm.)*	Calc fluor No 1	10
	Calc phos No 2	5
	Ferr phos No 4	15
	Kali phos No 6	5
	Nat mur No 9	5
	Silicea No 12	5
Stress; mental *(not for permanent use recommended)*	Ferr phos No 4	5
	Kali phos No 6	10
	Kali sulf No 7	
	Mag phos No 8	5
	Nat mur No 9	5
	Kali bromat No 14	3
Stress; physical	Calc phos No 2	5
	Ferr phos No 4	10
	Kali phos No 6	5
	Mag phos No 8	5
	Nat mur No 9	5
Stretch marks *(external use with similar Tissue Salts recomm.)*	Calc fluor No 1	10
	Kali phos No 6	5
	Nat mur No 9	5
	Silicea No 12	10
Struma; enlargement of the thyroid gland *(see GP)*	Calc fluor No 1	5
	Calc phos No 2	5
	Kali mur No 5	5
	Mag phos No 8	5
	Kali jodat No 15	10
Stye; eye, hordeolum	Calc sulf No 3	7
	Ferr phos No 4	20
	Kali mur No 5	10

	Nat phos No 10	7
	Silicea No 12	7
Sun burn; to restore the skin *(external use with similar Tissue Salts recomm.)*	Calc fluor No 1	5
	Ferr phos No 4	5
	Kali phos No 6	5
	Kali sulf No 7	5
	Nat mur No 9	10
	Silicea No 12	5
Suppuration *(external use with similar Tissue Salts recomm.)*	Calc sulf No 3	10
	Nat phos No 10	5
	Silicea No 12	3
Suppuration; gaping wound	Calc sulf No 3	10
Sweating; greasy	Nat phos No 10	10
Sweating; poor	Nat mur No 9	10
Sweating; tendency for sweats	Calc phos No 2	10
	Kali jodat No 15	5
Sweating; without any effort	Calc phos No 2	7
	Calc carbonic No 22	5
Sweating; bad smelling	Silicea No 12	7
Swelling; glands, soft	Kali mur No 5	10
Swollen hands, feet, legs	Nat sulf No 11	7

T

Tallow; disorders	Nat phos No 10	10
Taste; bitter	Nat sulf No 11	5
Taste; diminish or loss	Nat mur No 9	10
	Zincum mur No 21	5
Teeth; getting transparent	Calc fluor No 1	5
	Calc phos No 2	10
Teeth; looseness	Calc fluor No 1	7
Teething; children	Calc fluor No 1	5
	Ferr phos No 4	5
	Kali phos No 6	3
	Nat mur No 9	5
Temperament; Restlessness	Kali bromatum No 14	10
Tendon; shortening, Dupuytren's contracture *(external use with similar Tissue Salts recomm.)*	Calc fluor No 1	15
	Ferr phos No 4	7
	Kali phos No 6	5

	Mag phos No 8	5
	Nat mur No 9	5
	Nat phos No 10	5
	Silicea No 12	5
Tendon; lengthening	Calc fluor No 1	10
(external use with similar Tissue Salts recomm.)	Kali phos No 6	10
	Nat mur No 9	10
	Silicea No 12	5
Tendon; strain	Calc fluor No 1	10
(external use with similar Tissue Salts recomm.)	Calc phos No 2	5
	Ferr phos No 4	15
	Kali phos No 6	5
	Nat mur No 9	5
	Silicea No 12	5
Tendonitis	Ferr phos No 4	10
(external use with similar Tissue Salts recomm.)	Nat mur No 9	5
	Nat phos No 10	5
	Silicea No 12	5
Tennis elbow	Calc fluor No 1	5
(external use with similar Tissue Salts recomm.)	Calc phos No 2	10
	Ferr phos No 4	10
	Nat mur No 9	5
	Nat phos No 10	5
	Silicea No 12	5
Tension; neck, back, lumbar column	Calc fluor No 1	3
(external use with similar Tissue Salts recomm.)	Calc phos No 2	10
	Ferr phos No 4	7
	Nat mur No 9	5
	Nat phos No 10	10
	Silicea No 12	5
	Calc carbonic No 22	3
Thirst; intense	Nat mur No 9	10
Thirst; poor	Calc fluor No 1	5
	Nat mur No 9	10
Throat; clear the throat, convulsive	Kali jodat No 15	5
Throat; sore	Ferr phos No 4	10
	Kali mur No 5	3
	Nat phos No 10	5
Throat; sore, suppurate (Angina)	Calc sulph No 3	10
	Ferr phos No 4	10
	Kali mur No 5	5
	Nat phos No 10	7
Thyroid gland; hyperthyreose	Kali mur No 5	5
(See GP!)	Kali bromatum No 14	5
	Kali jodat No 15	5

	Lithium mur No 16	5
	Cuprum arsenic No 19	5
	Selenium No 26	5
Thyroid gland; hypothyreose *(See GP!)*	Kali bromatum No 14	5
	Kali jodat No 15	5
	Cuprum arsenic No 19	5
	Selenium No 26	5
Thrombosis *(see GP)*	Calc phos No 2	5
	Ferr phos No 4	5
	Kali mur No 5	10
	Kali phos No 6	5
	Nat mur No 9	5
	Nat phos No 10	5
	Nat sulf No 11	5
Thrombosis; prophylaxis of thrombosis (Airplane)	Ferr phos No 4	10
	Kali mur No 5	10
	Kali phos No 6	5
	Nat mur No 9	5
Tic nervous; mimic spasm (lid, labial angle)	Nat phos No 10	5
	Silicea No 12	7
Tingling; numbness sensation (hands, feet)	Calc phos No 2	7
Tiredness; due to exhaustion	Calc phos No 2	5
	Kali phos No 6	10
	Nat mur No 9	10
	Calc carbonic No 22	5
Tiredness; due to oxygen deficiency *(often in later afternoon)*	Ferr phos No 4	10
	Kali sulf No 7	5
	Nat sulf No 11	7
Tiredness; due to acidity *(check your diet!)*	Nat phos No 10	10
Tongue; coated vesicular	Nat mur No 9	5
Tongue; dry	Nat mur No 9	7
Tongue; fissured	Calc fluor No 1	3
Tongue; furred, coated brownish-yellow	Kali sulf No 7	7
Tongue; furred, coated greenish-yellow	Nat sulf No 11	7
Tongue; furred, coated whitish	Kali mur No 5	7
Tonsillitis	Calc sulf No 3	5
	Ferr phos No 4	7
	Kali mur No 5	5
	Nat phos No 10	5

Tonsillitis; pus-formation	Calc sulf No 3	10
	Nat phos No 10	5
	Silicea No 12	3
Toothache	Ferr phos No 4	7
	Kali phos No 6	3
	Kali sulf No 7	3
	Mag phos No 8	HOT 8*
	Nat mur No 9	3
Toothache during pregnancy	Calc fluor No 1	5
	Calc phos No 2	10
	Nat mur No 9	5
Travel sickness	Calc fluor No 1	5
	Calc phos No 2	5
	Ferr phos No 4	5
	Kali mur No 5	5
	Kali phos No 6	10
	Mag phos No 8	HOT 8*
	Nat phos No 10	5
Tuberculosis; TB	Calc phos No 2	10
(Additional to medical assistance)	Ferr phos No 4	5
	Kali mur No 5	5
	Mag phos No 8	5
	Nat mur No 9	5
Tuberculosis; TB with high fever	Calc phos No 2	10
(Additional to medical assistance)	Ferr phos No 4	5
	Kali mur No 5	5
	Kali phos No 6	10
	Mag phos No 8	5
	Nat mur No 9	5

U

Ulcer of the leg; Ulcus cruris	Calc sulf No 3	5
	Ferr phos No 4	10
	Kali mur No 5	5
	Kali phos No 6	5
	Nat sulf No 11	10
	Arsenum jodat No 24	3
Uric acid; high level	Nat phos No 10	10
	Silicea No 12	5
	Nat bicarbonic No 23	5
Uric acid; prevention calculus	Calc phos No 2	3
	Mag phos No 8	5
	Nat phos No 10	10
	Nat bicarbonic No 23	3
Urinary retention	Nat mur No 9	7
Urinary tract; inflammation	Calc sulf No 3	5

	Ferr phos No 4	10
	Nat mur No 9	5
	Nat phos No 10	5
	Lithium mur No 16	3
Urticaria; urticarial rash	Calc phos No 2	5
	Ferr phos No 4	5
	Kali mur No 5	5
	Kali phos No 6	5
	Mag phos No 8	5
	Nat mur No 9	5
	Nat sulf No 11	10

V

Vaccination; pre & after	Calc phos No 2	10
	Calc sulf No 3	10
	Ferr phos No 4	10
	Kali mur No 5	10
Vaccination; skin rash	Calc phos No 2	10
	Kali mur No 5	10
	Nat sulf No 11	10
Vagina; burning, tender	Kali sulf No 7	5
	Nat mur No 9	10
	Nat sulf No 11	5
	Zincum mur No 21	5
Vagina; itching and dry	Nat mur No 9	7
	Kali jodat No 15	3
Vagina: very dry mucous membranes	Kali phos No 6	5
	Nat mur No 9	10
	Nat phos No 10	5
	Zincum mur No 21	5
Varicose veins *(external use with similar Tissue Salts recomm.)*	Calc fluor No 1	5
	Kali mur No 5	5
	Nat phos No 10	10
	Silicea No 12	10
Varicose veins; prevention	Calc fluor No 1	5
	Kali mur No 5	5
	Mag phos No 8	5
	Nat phos No 10	10
	Silicea No 12	5
	Nat bicarbonic No 23	5
Varicose veins; bursting	Calc fluor No 1	10
	Silicea No 12	10
Varicose ulcer *(external use with similar Tissue Salts recomm.)*	Calc fluor No 1	5
	Kali mur No 5	5
	Nat phos No 10	5
	Nat sulf No 11	10

	Silicea No 12	5
Vein disorders	Calc fluor No 1	5
(external use with similar Tissue Salts recomm.)	Kali mur No 5	5
	Nat phos No 10	10
	Silicea No 12	5
Vertigo; old age	Calc Phos No 2	10
	Ferr phos No 4	10
	Kali phos No 6	10
	Mag phos No 8	HOT 8
	Nat sulf No 11	7
Vitiligo	Calc sulf No 3	5
	Kali mur No 5	5
	Kali sulf No 7	5
	Nat sulf No 11	10
* only if not thyroid related	Cuprum arsenic No 19*	5
Vomiting + purging; emetocatharsis	Ferr phos No 4	10
	Nat sulf No 11	10
Vomiting	Ferr phos No 4	5
(dissolve minerals in water, very small sips)	Kali phos No 6	5
	Kali sulf No 7	5
	Nat phos No 10	10
	Nat sulf No 11	10

W

Warts	Kali mur No 5	5
(also external use with paste of tissue salts)	Nat sulf No 11	5
Waste production, elimination	Nat sulf No 11	7
Weakness, in general	Calc phos No 2	5
	Ferr phos No 4	5
	Kali phos No 6	5
	Nat mur No 9	5
	Calc carbonic No 22	5
Weight loss; cure	Kali mur No 5	5
(30 min before or after a meal)	Kali sulf No 7	5
	Nat mur No 9	5
	Nat phos No 10	5
	Nat sulf No 11	5
Weight loss; unexpected	Calc phos No 2	5
(see GP!)	Kali phos No 6	10
	Nat mur No 9	10
	Silicea No 12	3
	Kali arsenic No 13	3
	Calc sulfur No 18	3
Worm infestation; ascaris, thread worm	Ferr phos No 4	5
	Kali phos No 6	5

	Kali sulf No 7	5
	Nat phos No 10	10
Wounds bleeding *(external use with similar Tissue Salts recomm.)*	Ferr phos No 4	10
Wrinkles; anti ageing	Calc fluor No 1	5
	Kali phos No 6	5
	Nat mur No 9	5
	Silicea No 12	10
	Calc bicarbonic No 22	5
Wrinkled skin; beauty remedy	Silicea No 12	10
	Calc carbonic No 22	10

Bibliography

Boericke William, M.D. & Dewey Willis A., M.D.: *Twelve Tissue Remedies of Schueßler*, 1888, reprinted 1972

Feichtinger Thomas / Mandl E. / Niedan-Feichtinger S.: *Handbuch der Biochemie nach Dr. Schüßler*, 1999

Feichtinger Thomas: *Psychosomatik und Biochemie nach Dr. Schüßler*, 2003

Feichtinger Thomas: *Antlitzanalyse in der Biochemie nach Dr. Schüßler*, 2002

Hickethier, K.: Sonnerschau – *Lehrbuch der Anlitzdiagnostik*, 1984

Prevenhueber von, Alice: *Mineral Replacement*

Schüßler WH: *Eine abgekürzte Therapie. Anleitung zur biochemischen Behandlung der Krankheiten. 31. Aufl. Oldenburg und Leipzig*, 1904

Taggart Mc, Lynne: *What doctors don't tell you*, 1996

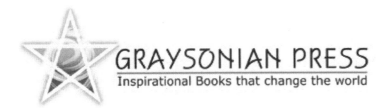

To view books of inspiration visit www.graysonian.com Or contact: pat@graysonian.com
Tel +27 11 6462956
PO Box 47062, Parklands, South Africa, 2121

Workshops and consultations

Eva conducts:

- Seminars 'Junior Facial Analysis'
- On site workshops/demonstrations for health shops, pharmacies, naturalpaths, etc
- Introductory workshops 'Tissue Salts and Facial Signs'
- Presentations to corporate, coffee groups, lunches, groups of interested people (e.g. Sports clubs, customers of a shop, homoeopaths)

All presentations are based on Eva's writings.

To contact Eva +27 076 819 4590 or email info@facialanalysis.co.za